CHOO
WHEELCHAIR

A Guide for Optimal Independence

CHOOSING A WHEELCHAIR

A Guide for Optimal Independence

Gary Karp

O'REILLY™

Cambridge • Köln • Paris • Sebastopol • Tokyo

Choosing a Wheelchair: A Guide for Optimal Independence
by Gary Karp

Published by O'Reilly & Associates, Inc., 101 Morris Street, Sebastopol, CA 95472.

Series Editor: Linda Lamb

Editor: Carol Wenmoth

Production Editor: Claire Cloutier LeBlanc

Printing History:

July 1998:   First Edition

Table of Contents

Introduction

CHOOSING A WHEELCHAIR is not an especially pleasant process, particularly if you are facing it for the first time. You—or someone you love—might need a wheelchair because of a recent traumatic injury or illness. You might be going through a time of grief and deep emotion. Sad or angry feelings might be stirred up by the very notion of choosing a wheelchair. You might anticipate that you will recover from your injury or illness, and think a personalized wheelchair isn't necessary. But the right wheelchair is a liberator, not a prison. When you choose the right chair, your quality of life increases dramatically. Even people with severe disabilities can have a considerable degree of independence and activity with the right wheels. For those who no longer need it at some point, having had the right chair will mean better health and greater strength.

Perhaps you're an experienced rider who needs some new wheels. There are probably a lot of choices and options that didn't exist when you got your current chair, and you want to make sure you take full advantage of new features and designs. Maybe your therapist or dealer could have done a better job before, and, now that you have learned from using your present chair, you want to ensure that you get the best chair possible this time.

Wheelchair design has advanced tremendously in just the last decade. No longer limited to the aluminum folding chairs you might be accustomed to seeing in hospitals or airports, there is now a huge array of designs and options for both manual and power wheelchairs. Wheelchairs are highly adjustable—or custom built—available in various sizes, with features to make driving them easier, safer, and more dignified.

Modern chairs are also better looking; even power chairs have become less bulky and obtrusive. There has been much effort to reduce the visual emphasis on the disability, and to bring more attention to the person. Thanks to a growing population of active wheelchair users who have no desire to stay at home or sit in institutions, there are great demands on the wheelchair industry. Because of this growing market, manufacturers can now justify continuing advanced design efforts to help people continue their lives with the greatest possible independence and activity.

This book will help you understand more about what a wheelchair is these days, and prepare you for the process of identifying the right one. Detailed information about all the features of a wheelchair, and how each contributes to optimal mobility and comfort, will help you be an informed decision-maker.

This book also covers funding issues, maintenance, and wheeling style. At the end of the book is a list of resources to help you locate the best chair for you, as well as suggestions for further reading.

This book will make choosing a wheelchair easier, and enable you to emerge from the process with a chair that truly meets your needs.

CHAPTER ONE

The Wheelchair Revolution

You've seen the old chairs in movies—remember the wheelchair used by the evil Mr. Potter in Jimmy Stewart's *It's a Wonderful Life*? Early wheelchairs were made of wood, had tall backs, and were very wide and heavy. The wheels were not easily pushed by the rider—if they could be at all. The design assumed that the chair's occupant would always need help. These chairs could not be folded, and were too bulky even for the huge trunks of early model cars. The other image associated with the old-fashioned wheelchair was the obligatory blanket hanging over the lap, a feature naturally bestowed upon Mr. Potter.

The idea of a wheelchair for an active person used to be a foreign concept. But wheelchairs aren't what they used to be. Even in the last ten years, tremendous improvements have been made. Today's chairs offer variety, flexibility, greater physical comfort, and independence. They also take into consideration the many different lifestyles and physical needs of riders, as well as their right to ride with dignity.

It's worthwhile to have some sense of the evolution of wheelchair design, which has been inevitably tied to changes in technology and in the way our culture views people with disabilities. As you go through the process of selecting your chair, you might find it helpful to know something about the forces and personalities that brought about the tremendous improvements in wheelchair design. It's an interesting and remarkable story. This chapter gives an overview of the wheelchair revolution, and some of the innovative people who made it happen.

Development of modern chairs

In 1918, Herbert Everest became a paraplegic in a mining accident. After years of frustration with the limitations of the "Mr. Potter chair," he asked his engineer friend, Harry Jennings, to design a less bulky, more convenient wheelchair. In 1932, Jennings built the first folding wheelchair, feather-light for its day at a mere fifty-five pounds. The two friends proceeded to establish Everest & Jennings, the company that for many years would hold a near monopoly of the wheelchair market. The company's position in the market was so strong that they were ultimately forced to settle an antitrust suit brought by the Department of Justice charging that they set wheelchair prices artificially high.

> My first two chairs were E & J. There was really no other choice. At the time, they were state of the art, using lighter aluminum, in a narrow adult design with options like pneumatic tires, swingaway footrests, and removable armrests.

In the 1960s, things began to change. One of the first people to experiment with a different design than the traditional Everest & Jennings chair was Bud Rumpel, a machinist with polio who built a custom wheelchair for sports use. Bob Hall of New Hall's Wheels in Cambridge, Massachusetts, was an early pioneer in racing and sport chairs. He comments:

> I believe wheelchair design has stemmed from sports. That is where the real innovation came from. Some of us went with servicing individuals, others went for larger production.

The first attempt at a new commercial product came from a company called Quadra, which experimented for the first time with even lighter-weight metal alloys, square frame members, quick-release wheels, and color choices.

But it was another innovator who began producing lightweight designs in volume and mass marketing them. In 1978, Marilyn Hamilton crashed her hang glider and became a spinal cord injured paraplegic. Like Everest before her, she was frustrated by the existing options she found for wheelchairs. She wanted to play tennis, and knew enough about design from her hang gliding experience to realize that the E & J chair was outmoded. There was room for improvement using modern materials. Even more important, there was a more evolved attitude about what kind of life was possible with a disability, but no equipment to accommodate it. Although not the first to explore these issues, she ultimately scored the biggest success.

Just as Everest asked Jennings, Hamilton asked friends Don Helman and Jim Okamoto—who had experience building hang gliders—to design an ultralight wheelchair. They took the weight of the chair down to twenty-six pounds from the standard fifty-five. It sported a light-blue frame, a lower back, and a more refined, stylish look. The Quickie Designs wheelchair company was born.

> My new Quickie chair was twenty pounds lighter than my previous E & J chair. The light weight made it easier to lift the chair in and out of the car, for friends to carry me up and down stairs. People still react to the new chair, sensing its lightweight design. I often lift off one of my footrests and hand it to them to demonstrate how light it is. Once the footrest is in their grasp, they're usually amazed.

This revolution in wheelchair design took the Everest & Jennings company by surprise. By the 1980s, they no longer had disabled managers to guide them, and had lost touch with the needs of their customers. Much to their chagrin, Everest & Jennings found themselves losing $88 million between 1989 and 1991, because they had rested on their laurels and neglected to refine their products.

E & J is still on the scene, with a selection of advanced lightweight, fixed-frame chairs in their catalog, but without the position they held for so long—and might have maintained with a little foresight.

But they are not likely to disappear, either, as they evidently have recognized their error and are once again offering competitive, advanced designs.

Meanwhile, the Quickie chair was widely adopted as the norm, as people flocked to its lighter weight, less institutional-looking design, and sometimes wild choice of colors—including bright, fluorescent colors and patterns, or what Hamilton called the "screaming neon chair." The Quickie design can even be credited with nurturing the disabled civil rights movement, not only because riders were able to achieve greater independence with the new chairs, but because their self-image was unburdened of the institutional feel of the older design. The world saw more of the person, less of the chair. The sight of wheelchair users in public became more common, beginning the process of a shifting public awareness of disability. With the wheelchair less of an obstacle to independence, the remaining obstacles—in the realms of politics and culture—could be faced. Joseph Shapiro writes in his book, *No Pity*:

> *Hamilton had reinvented the wheelchair. She took a piece of medical equipment and made it fun and sporty. She took the universal symbol of sickness and turned it into a symbol of disability self-pride.*

The updated, enlightened design of the Quickie chair helped to create a dramatic change in the way people thought about wheelchairs:

> *After I finally made the switch to my first Quickie II in 1989, I visited friends in Los Angeles. When Richard saw the new wheels, he called out to his wife, "Hey, Pat! Gary's got a designer wheelchair!" His conception of the wheelchair had been rocked, a paradigm broken.*

At the same time that the wheelchair was being reinvented, there was also a continuing evolution in wheelchair cushion design. Cushions had become lighter as well as better looking and more effective. Better cushions contributed to the overall improvement in chair comfort and reduction of weight. They also allowed people to spend many more hours in their chairs without as much risk of pressure sores. Able to spend more time in their wheelchairs, riders found new possibilities for education, employment, fun, and travel.

Power chairs

The next frontier was the power wheelchair. (Power chairs are no longer referred to as "electric chairs," for obvious reasons.) Like manual chairs, power chairs have come a long way since the first models. Early power chairs were typically bulky affairs, essentially a manual chair with a motor, batteries, and drive mechanism added on. Slow, clumsy to handle, challenged by hills, and difficult or impossible to transport in a car, they could be severely limiting, although they provided more mobility to those unable to push a manual chair.

Today's power chairs have been redesigned from the ground up—fully integrated, smooth, powerful, and loaded with options that allow people with more severe disabilities to be more active than ever before possible.

Once again, Marilyn Hamilton played the role of innovator, unfortunately as a result of an auto accident which broke her legs and wrists. This time it was the power chair that failed to meet her test. The Quickie P200 was introduced under the banner of Motion Designs, soon to be purchased by Sunrise Medical. The P200 is much lighter and more attractive than the old power chairs. It is also capable of being broken down to its components for storage in the trunk of a car and ease of maintenance. Modular design would revolutionize power chair design and manufacturing. (Invacare has also been influential in the research and development of the modular power chair, including the use of separate motors and suspension.)

Wheelchair manufacturer Permobil subsequently introduced the ChairMan Corpus model with a remarkable array of features, all controllable by the user. The back can tilt to relieve pressure on the spine and sit bones, crucial for power chair users who are unable to lift themselves with their arms. The seat and footrests can also be tilted and elevated. It is even possible to be raised to a standing position in some of their models. The design includes shock absorbers and front-wheel direct drive.

The continuing evolution of the wheelchair

Wheelchair producers have proliferated in recent years. Not even Quickie holds a monopoly such as the one formerly enjoyed by Everest & Jennings. Companies such as Colours, Permobil, Otto Bock, and Invacare are only a few of the more widely recognized providers of wheelchairs. All these companies must work harder—and at a faster pace—at development and innovation to maintain their share of the market.

Wheelchairs have gotten much more complex. Many chairs now use an adjustable plate for the wheels; this allows adjustment of the axle position in relation to the frame, both vertically and horizontally. The height and angle of the front casters can be customized, as well as the height of the back, and sometimes the angle of the seat pan. Thanks to the immense recent evolution in design and manufacture, there is a chair out there that can accommodate your particular physical condition in a way that offers you a level of activity and independence that is unique in our human history. Even people with what would be considered severe disabilities can participate in ways that were previously impossible.

At the same time, certain niches have appeared, such as athletic chairs for racing, rugby, and tennis. Then there's the unique Iron Horse chair, whose advertisements show someone waist-deep in a river while fly-fishing from his wheelchair. More than ever there are small companies offering specialized designs, or offering what they believe to be the next great innovation in chair design.

The tradition of necessity as the mother of invention continues. The Falcon High Rider was developed by Tom Houston, a pipe fitter who wanted to get back to the work he had always done. He wanted a chair he could still drive in a standing position, and could get through tight spaces. Similarly, the OmegaTrac from Teftec was developed by a father and son engineering team for the quadriplegic son who needed to traverse rough terrain.

Ralf Hotchkiss, an engineer and paraplegic chair user, took an entirely different approach when he set out to build his own chair. Hotchkiss not only wanted a better chair, but was concerned about the high prices and maintenance problems of commercial wheelchairs. He also wanted to focus on third-world countries, where thousands of people are trapped without mobility. Hotchkiss joined with others to develop the Whirlwind chair, which can be made with local materials found in poor countries for vastly less money than it takes to buy an American chair. The design is truly collaborative; many people contributed ideas for such details as wheel bearings and frame components. Now head of the Wheeled Mobility Center at San Francisco State University, and the recipient of a MacArthur Foundation Genius Grant, Hotchkiss and company have traveled around the world, training hundreds of people and helping them set up shops to produce the Whirlwind chair locally.

There are some concerns about the future progress of the wheelchair industry. As with the computer software and automotive industries, wheelchair production is concentrating into the hands of a few large producers, with an array of specialty products from smaller companies.

Large companies like Quickie and Invacare have become purchasers of wheelchair technology. Small producers, who tend to push the limits and test the boundaries of wheelchair design and development, often find it makes more business sense to sell their innovations to one of the large manufacturers than to try to build a profitable organization of their own.

Karl Ylonen of Care Corporation in Vancouver, Washington, has mixed feelings about this trend. He has been selling wheelchairs for more than ten years and is concerned that the industry "is concentrating on big suppliers and it might limit innovation. I feel a responsibility to give my clients a choice, and I don't want to put all my eggs in one basket. We need small as well as large producers."

One hopes that the wheelchair industry will not forget the tough lesson learned by Everest & Jennings, who lost so much business to the small upstart of Quickie. (Some fear that now even Quickie is resting on its laurels.) Then again, one could say that E & J so horribly ignored the obvious need for streamlined design and the use of new materials that they left the door open for someone to do exactly what Marilyn Hamilton and her team did at Quickie. It's hard to imagine a company repeating that mistake—much less monopolizing the market—in this new competitive environment.

CHAPTER TWO

Large Versus Small Manufacturers

LIKE OTHER MANUFACTURERS, wheelchair producers come in many varieties. There are large corporate wheelchair manufacturers, small specialized producers, and innovative new companies hoping to make a name for themselves. Naturally, you will want to find out what various companies offer before deciding which manufacturer produces the optimum chair for you. Your therapist and the dealer with whom you work will have a lot of information about the major producers, and hopefully between the two of them, they will also have a well-rounded knowledge of smaller producers.

No one can know it all, however, so it will be up to you to do some investigating on your own. This chapter will discuss the major advantages offered by the large companies, alert you to some pitfalls, and suggest reasons why it might be well worth the time and effort to explore the products offered by small or relatively new companies.

Advantages of major manufacturers

As you begin shopping for the right chair, you will soon hear the names of the largest manufacturers of wheelchairs and accessories: Invacare, Everest & Jennings, Quickie Designs, and Permobil. These large companies employ hundreds of people, and some are owned by parent companies with considerable financial resources.

Greater resources mean major wheelchair manufacturers can invest more in research and development than their smaller competitors. They can afford to build many prototypes, and can take a little longer to develop new designs since these large firms have a steadier stream of revenue from existing products.

Larger companies can afford to spend time and money on aesthetics. They hire industrial designers to work with mechanical engineers to make attractive designs that also meet functional and manufacturing criteria (achieving varying levels of success, depending on whom you ask). Of course, just because a chair looks better doesn't mean it is better, but aesthetics are not irrelevant. If you are a person who is fashion conscious, affected by your sense of how you present yourself stylistically to the world, aesthetics are a very real consideration that is not to be minimized.

Following are additional advantages offered by large wheelchair manufacturers:

- They have comprehensive lines of wheelchair products, with plenty of options and accessories.

- They have been in the business long enough to have a lot of experience behind them.

- They have refined their manufacturing and design over those years, and will probably be around for the foreseeable future.

- They are reputable, and generally make good chairs, assuming you select the right model, properly configured.

- Your dealer will have more experience maintaining and repairing chairs from larger manufacturers.

Some would also argue that finding parts and service away from home is easier when your chair is made by one of the large firms, although the very complexity and vast array of options from the large producers make it impossible for dealers to carry all parts for all chairs. Whether you travel or stay at home, you are likely to have to wait for a part to be shipped. If you travel often, availability of parts is definitely something to ask about before deciding to purchase.

One woman who is shopping for a new power chair has learned the hard way how important it is to consider servicing issues:

> When choosing a new chair, the biggest single consideration for me will be servicing. The closest repair person for my current chair is three hours away. They don't come into my town but once every other week, and they do not have a loaner while mine is down. This time I will purchase a chair that can be serviced locally from a dealer who can provide a loaner should mine go down for more than a few hours. Since this is a very small rural town and there is only one business here that sells power chairs, my choice(s) will be limited to either whatever they can service or a chair that has a reputation for not breaking down. I wish someone had talked to me about servicing when I purchased my first power chair.

Don't choose a large manufacturer too quickly

The same resources that allow large companies to offer you a wide selection also mean they have more money for advertising and marketing. It is easier for them to get exposure through magazines and trade shows. They are able to sell more chairs, often at higher prices, so they can offer dealers more profit, which encourages dealers to recommend those chairs. In other words, the major manufacturers have all of the usual advantages of large companies in any competitive marketplace, and it is easy for consumers to assume these big names must be the best choice.

Not everyone agrees. Some people believe that the large producers are not putting enough priority on the individual. Jeff Ewing of Falcon Rehabilitation in Commerce City, Colorado, says:

> We're trying to stay away from what we feel some of our competitors are doing—trying to sell as many chairs as they can. They don't concern themselves enough with whether it's what the person really needs.

This is not to say that the large producers don't care, or that they don't have equally supportive people on their staff. Some large wheelchair makers have on-staff therapists who work with customers to ensure they get the right wheels. These therapists know there will be some customers for whom their company doesn't have an appropriate chair, and in those cases the customer should be referred to another manufacturer.

Obviously, a lot depends on the individuals helping you choose your chair, but it's a good idea to be aware that dealers and salespeople might have more incentive to sell you a chair from one of the large manufacturers. Even if higher profits don't come into the picture, there are other reasons why a dealer may focus on chairs from the major producers, overlooking a potentially more appropriate product from a smaller company. For instance, a dealer might not be aware of a particular model of chair. And if dealers shared everything they knew, it would probably overwhelm the customer. Karl Ylonen of Care Corporation agrees:

> If I were to bring all of my product information with me when I go out to meet a customer, I would have to carry four file drawers and a shelf unit, and even then it wouldn't cover everything!

It's equally unrealistic to expect therapists to have all the answers. Jeff Ewing of Falcon offers this advice:

> Therapists tend to be used to dealing with the large suppliers. People need to do their own research to find what's best for them, and not always accept what's being recommended just because the therapist or dealer says so. It's natural for therapists and dealers to suggest what they know, and they only have so much time to learn everything that's out there.

Be aware that if you decide on a chair from a major manufacturer, you may have to wait longer for delivery. There are many stories of large producers having a tough time delivering their chairs quickly. You could wait months for some of the more popular designs, particularly power chairs. You are likely to have waited a long time already—working with therapists and dealers, trying out demonstration chairs, perhaps struggling with insurers or bureaucrats to get coverage. If you have a pressing need to have a chair by a certain date, this could affect a choice between two competing options. Then again, getting the chair you really need is important enough that it behooves you to be as patient as possible.

Your dealer should check with the suppliers of the chairs you are considering to give you their current production schedule.

Find out what small manufacturers offer

There are dozens of small companies out there making wheelchairs. Since they don't have the marketing budgets of the big firms, you might not hear about them. (See the *Resources* section at the end of this book for a comprehensive listing of manufacturers.) It is very difficult for dealers to represent every option in the world, so it is a challenge for the smaller makers to reach you, to let you know if they are the best solution. They know they have to work a little harder and try different strategies to get your attention.

However, if you decide a small producer's chair is the right one for you, your dealer should be perfectly willing to call the manufacturer and ask them to sell you one.

Bob Hall of New Hall's Wheels prefers to sell directly to customers:

Our basic strategy is direct sales. The dealers are pretty much going to push the products that they make the greater profit from. Our customers can either deal with us directly or work with the dealer. Sometimes working with the dealer is what's most convenient for the user, so we do that. We'll get them a chair either way, but we can't provide the kinds of discounts [to dealers] typically found in the health care market. So selling direct to the customer works well for us.

Hall is not concerned about being swallowed up by or having to compete with the large producers. "I don't feel like I'm competing with anybody but myself to create a better product."

The emphasis on making better, innovative products—or specialized ones—is a recurrent theme among small manufacturers, as is offering more personalized service. Says Jeff Ewing:

> We're not in this business as much for the money as to help people out. Of course, like any business, you need enough money to keep it going. But we're not that concerned with producing mass numbers of these chairs. We'd rather focus on a small group and help them out to the best of our abilities.

Many of the smaller suppliers have no desire to knock down a Goliath. They fill niches, meeting the needs of smaller populations. For example, Wheelcare, Inc., of Camarillo, California, makes the PowerChair, a motorized wheelchair that would never be used by a high-level quadriplegic person. It is designed for people who've had a stroke, elderly riders who might be in a temporary recovery, or people with multiple sclerosis during an exacerbation, for example. The PowerChair is a very basic, aluminum chair with limited adjustability. Its trick is the use of motors outside of the wheels, using a friction drive rather than gears or belts. The design allows the chair to be folded to thirteen inches without removing anything, including the batteries. It can also change quickly between manual and power with the flick of a switch. Wheelcare has already developed its drive package as an accessory to models from Everest & Jennings and Invacare. This is clearly their little corner of the market.

Many small producers customize each chair, building it exactly to order. Some noteworthy examples follow.

- The HiRider from Falcon Rehabilitation is a power chair that can stand you up. Says Falcon's Jeff Ewing, "We get detailed information about the person, and the chair is built to their height, weight, back height, seat depth, and so on. It's not a standard chair. We don't have them sitting on the shelf." The HiRider is popular with golfers. Falcon offers optional wheels that won't damage the grass, and a hookup that allows the chair to be towed by a golf cart to preserve battery power, as well as many other options.

- The Champion chair from Paraglide Medical in Florida was designed by paraplegic racecar driver Bill Joule. It is a lightweight (less than 20 pounds), rigid-frame chair that is made by hand.

- The Iron Horse was designed by George Duffy, who became a T-9 spinal cord paraplegic in 1969. An avid outdoorsman, Duffy found he broke a standard wheelchair every two years, and finally got fed up enough to build one of his own. The custom-built frames of the Iron Horse have a lifetime guarantee. Duffy was the first ever to put independent suspension on a wheelchair. In 1998, Iron Horse introduced their first power chair.

- The Hallmark chair from New Hall's Wheels is a rigid-frame, brushed-aluminum chair that is very minimal and elegant in its design. It is also extremely lightweight, at only 19 pounds. It is custom built without much of the usual adjustability you find in other chairs. Bob Hall explains, "We have a system of getting all the dimensions of the user. We understand their needs, so we build it right in the first place. Then they don't need all that extra adjustable hardware. It only weighs more and requires more maintenance." New Hall's Wheels began by making racing chairs in the late 1970s. Their original Road Hugger wheelchair is on permanent display at New York's Museum of Modern Art. They have even advertised it in nondisability publications like GQ and Glamour magazines. Aesthetics and performance are high priorities.

- Wheelchairs of Kansas makes a manual and a power chair that will hold a person up to 600 pounds in weight. It comes in widths of up to 26 inches.

- 21st Century Scientific also makes a wide chair called the Bounder, which can be customized to almost any dimension for users who weigh up to 700 pounds.

As you can see, there is a lot to be learned by exploring the smaller wheelchair producers. Following are the most important benefits offered by small companies, including those that are newer to the industry.

- They are generally passionate about their work, concerned with quality, and interested in helping people.

- You are likely to get more personal attention.

- You might find a chair that more specifically meets your needs, even one that can be more aggressively customized for you.

- Since smaller producers don't have huge production schedules, they may be able to deliver your chair faster than a large company.

- You might be able to find a better price.

One issue you will want to consider before deciding to purchase from a small producer is how important the look of your chair is to you. Wheelchairs designed by the smaller companies often tend to look like they were designed by an engineer, whose concerns are wholly functional, and whose training does not include aesthetics. Engineers are interested in the operation of the chair, and the ease of manufacturing it. This is not universally true of small producers, but is more the rule than the exception. (Two small companies notable for the aesthetic aspects of their products are Paraglide and New Hall's Wheels.)

If you are the personality type who is practical and unconcerned with flash or looking hip, a chair that looks like it was designed by an engineer is no problem for you. In fact, it might be the better chair. However, if you are concerned with appearance, be sure to ask about this.

You will also want to ask about the ease of finding service and getting parts for a chair made by a small manufacturer. Some small producers have simplified their designs specifically to reduce maintenance demands (as well as their own inventory costs). And some stay well stocked, so a part can be ordered quickly and sent to you.

You can also find ways to minimize service problems on the road. For instance, you can bring spare parts with you. In his book, *Moving Violations*, paraplegic journalist John Hockenberry describes his travels to Israel, where he was assigned as a reporter:

> I had brought two extra wheelchairs, an enormous box of parts, and three additional sets of wheels. There were two dozen tire patch kits, three sets of all-terrain tires, a heavy-duty drill, and a set of tools which apparently fit the airport X-ray profile of a grenade launcher!

Well, perhaps you wouldn't need to get quite that carried away, but you don't necessarily need to choose a large producer's chair when you can carry tubes, a small air pump, and a simple toolkit when you travel. It's also a good idea to have your chair checked out and well maintained before going on a trip—just as you would with your car or van—to avoid being stuck needing a part. That's an inconvenience no matter where you are or what you are riding in.

CHAPTER THREE

Who Pays for Your Chair?

THE QUALITY OF YOUR LIFE depends on getting the best and most appropriate wheels for your needs. This is not an area where it makes sense to skimp. Wheelchairs are very expensive. A typical manual chair can cost about $2,000. A fully equipped power chair can reach prices in the range of $30,000, although they generally will be closer to $10,000.

Because you need the best chair and it costs a lot, you have little choice but to rely on outside payers. Your chair might be paid for by a small or large insurance company, managed care such as a health maintenance organization (HMO) or planned provider organization (PPO), a government agency such as Vocational Rehabilitation or the Veterans Administration (VA), or a government plan like Medicare from the federal government or Medicaid from state government.

Whether private or public, funders are all conscious of their budgets and have a lot of motivation to limit their costs. In the recent environment of political pressure to control health care costs, it is becoming increasingly difficult to get approval for your ideal wheels, although this depends on exactly who is paying.

This chapter looks at the need to advocate for yourself, what issues might arise with various insurers, and sources for alternative funding.

Advocate for yourself

You need to be serious about being your own advocate when buying a wheelchair. Read your policies and contracts. Don't be afraid to ask questions or to make phone calls to find out what you need to know. Insurance companies and government agencies are bound under certain laws to give you information. It is indeed unfortunate that you should ever have to fight for what you are entitled to, but if it will make a difference in your health and quality of life, you should not hesitate to be persistent—just be well informed and reasonable at the same time.

There is no reason you can't question a policy that you consider inappropriate or unfair. The worst your funder can do is say no. But if you can make a good case, you just might be able to convince an insurer to reconsider. Dr. Michael Boninger, executive director of the Center for Assistive Technology at the University of Pittsburgh, specifies chairs for people. He advises, "If your policy only allows you a $200 wheelchair, then challenge it. If you fight hard enough, you might get the insurer to make an exception."

If you are unable to deal with funding problems, perhaps a family member, friend, case manager, or social worker would be willing to invest the effort to overcome resistance you might encounter from payers. Many local independent living centers offer advice or active assistance with funding issues.

While you will want to first exhaust all the normal avenues—discussed throughout this chapter—for overcoming a denial of funding, as a last resort you can take your case public. Local television or newspaper reporters might be interested in reporting about a funder who is denying coverage for clearly needed equipment. Funders don't like negative publicity, so they might be persuaded to do the right thing. Even if you still don't get funding, the report could flush out other forms of help such as a generous donor or someone with a used chair that meets your needs.

Funding agencies and organizations generally do not think proactively. They tend to resist paying for something now, even if it will prevent problems—and save money—later. For example, an insurer might not want to pay for a contoured back to help control the trunk of a rider's body. Contoured backs can reach prices of up to $800, but their use can prevent the need for more expensive equipment or corrective surgery later on.

Jody Greenhalgh, O.T.R., is an occupational therapist with UCSF/Stanford Rehabilitation Services in Stanford, California. She is closely involved in specifying wheelchairs for people. More than once, she has encountered someone with pressure-sore problems who has had an expensive surgery. She finds that often these problems could have been avoided if the person had been provided with a better wheelchair and positioning system in the first place.

> *We see patients who have severe skin ulcers. They've been on bed rest for months. A specialized wheelchair is medically recommended but denied by the insurer. The patient then requires a $50,000 surgery, after which he returns to the inadequate wheelchair. This causes the surgery to fail and pressure sores recur. The patient has to go back on long-term bed rest and repeat hospitalization.*

> *The insurance companies seem to be short-sighted, preferring to spend money on surgical intervention rather than paying for the right cushion and specialized wheelchair—which would ultimately save dollars and help the patient return to a productive and independent life.*

You might need to enlist the help of your physician, occupational or physical therapist, or other medical professional. The initial wheelchair prescription typically includes a "certificate of medical necessity," which is signed by the physician. If your funder denies the chair specified on your prescription, ask for help from your medical team. Your doctor or therapist can write to your funder, explaining in detail why that particular chair is medically necessary for you. Greenhalgh is an experienced advocate:

> I will write a lengthier justification if a wheelchair prescription is denied. Sometimes I pull up old cases to use as examples and say, "Look, we saved money by doing this." If I persevere it really does pay off, but the process can extend for months. It means I have to spend a lot of time on the phone and paperwork rather than treating patients.

It makes sense that when you are shopping for insurance, it is crucial to ask specific questions and look for the parts of the policy that address durable medical equipment (DME). Select your coverage wisely.

Another way you can help yourself is to research a wide variety of manufacturers. For instance, smaller producers are very aware of the need to increase business by making their products a more attractive option to funding sources, so they try to offer good solutions at lower costs. If you can find a less expensive solution to your needs by doing this kind of research, it might reduce complications in dealing with your funding source, and make it easier for you to get approval.

The contact person

The person you work with to get funding for your chair will depend on your funding source. For example, if your health coverage is from an insurance company, you might be dealing directly with an adjuster. Your contact person may not have much power to make independent decisions. Her job will be to apply the company/agency policies to each case, to follow the rules. She will probably have quite a load of cases, so it will be literally impossible for her to learn much about you, to remember the details of your case, or to take time to do much research into your needs. Her training is focused on the process of doing the work—which forms to use, what is covered and what is not, and who has what authority. Medical training is often limited, so, although she may have been taught some things about medical equipment, she probably will not be well versed in the details of wheelchair selection.

Not everyone will fit this model, but you will want to get to know your contact person, and do your best to understand her background. You don't want to make an enemy of this person, if you can help it. She has a lot of influence over your life. At the same time, she might represent an obstacle to getting what you need, and it may be necessary to speak to a supervisor in order to make sure all possibilities have been explored.

It is increasingly common for insurance companies and funding agencies to assign your file to a case manager. The case manager should be your advocate, putting your medical interests first above all. He may or may not be a nurse, or otherwise medically experienced. Your case manager will talk with doctors and therapists, confirm the policies and limits of your coverage, shop for the best prices (which is part of what makes case managers appealing to the insurer), and even contact social workers to seek out additional sources of funding or equipment if the policy does not cover you.

Sometimes case managers are on staff, or the insurer might have a contract with an outside provider of these services. If there is not a case manager assigned to you, ask for one. You do not have a legal right to a case manager, but it's likely your request will be granted, especially if you are pleasantly persistent. If possible, try to get a case manager with specific background in rehabilitation equipment and your specific disability.

Private insurance

There is a tendency to vilify insurance companies—rightfully so in some cases—but keep in mind that, in order to keep your premiums low and stay in business, insurers must control the costs of what they provide to you and other policy holders. You will be looking to get what you need so that you can live a full and comfortable life; your insurance company will be looking to place limits on what you get. Insurers also need to guard against the possibility that an unscrupulous wheelchair vendor might try to charge unnecessarily high prices in the belief that the "rich insurance company" has deep pockets.

Although you may have to assert yourself to get the right wheelchair, it's possible that approval from your insurance company will go smoothly. If your policy covers a wheelchair, the need for the prescribed chair is clear, and your vendor states a fair price, your insurance carrier might pay with little or no resistance.

Don't assume your insurance policy won't cover something you need. It's worth the effort to check your policy or discuss your situation with your insurance contact person. For example, insurers might well be willing to cover the cost of a new chair assuming you have a justifiable medical need.

I spent more years in my heavy E & J hospital-style wheelchair than I needed to, as it turned out. I was assuming, mistakenly, that my private insurance through my job would not pay for a new wheelchair. Even though people were telling me that I should get out of my old "tank" in favor of a new lightweight chair, I never did the research. I figured when the day arrived when I would have to replace my old wheels, I would have to pay for it myself.

Finally I made the call and discovered that my policy did indeed cover the cost of a wheelchair at least once in the life of the policy. They would pay 80 percent, and I could easily handle the difference. So I made the appointment with my rehab doctor, who approved a consultation with the occupational therapist, who referred me to the local dealer, and I had my first Quickie wheelchair.

Increasingly, private health coverage is being provided by managed care organizations rather than traditional insurance companies. Managed care organizations are extremely cost conscious. Some clients are finding it difficult to convince their HMO or PPO to buy them the wheelchair they really need. The ease with which you will be able to get the optimal chair for you depends on the fine print in the managed care plan, so before you enroll in such a program, be certain to understand their spending policies.

Jody Greenhalgh, of UCSF/Stanford Rehabilitation Services, has found that it is more difficult to get payment for more sophisticated chairs and positioning systems under managed care.

Managed care is following the Medicare model, using ceilings. HMOs often will just not pay for expensive equipment. Typically, they'll only pay for a low-end wheelchair. I try to make the case that it is not only a cost decision, but a medical decision.

If you already belong to a managed care plan, and they refuse to provide you with the chair you need, there are a number of things you can do to get your plan administrator to reconsider. First, ask your doctor or therapist to write a letter explaining why specific options are medically necessary. If they are unable to convince the administrator that a particular chair is essential for your health, you can appeal the decision. Most, if not all, HMOs and PPOs have a procedure for appeals and are required to give you information about how it works. Depending on your situation, you can persist further by enlisting the help of your employer's benefits department (if the coverage is employer-provided), writing to the state insurance commissioner, contacting an appropriate advocacy group, or appealing to your congressional representatives.

Medicare and Medicaid

Doe Cayting, co-founder of Wheelchairs of Berkeley, California, says that as a supplier she used to be able to concentrate on what was the best chair for the person, and funding was a side issue. These days, Cayting is concerned that Medicare ceilings are having too much influence on the design of chairs.

Very often now it is the funding that is driving the wheelchair selection. How Congress funds Medicare has a lot to do with it. If they want to sell chairs, the manufacturers have to make a chair

that Medicare is willing to pay for. I'm concerned that this is hav-
ing the effect of lowering the standards for chair design.

Medicare has established very specific ceilings for what it is willing to pay for a wheelchair. Unfortunately, it is usually an amount far lower than what your ideal chair will cost, particularly from a dealer who invests a lot of time in identifying the right chair, supplying you with trial chairs, and working hard to get it configured for you when it arrives. As of this writing, Medicare will not even let you pay additional money to make up the difference, although legislative efforts are trying to change this. You must accept the chair they are willing to buy, or they will not cover you.

People covered by state-funded Medicaid can face an even more serious problem—not being able to get any wheelchair. Cayting explains:

State government Medicaid programs treat wheelchairs as
optional equipment, and may or may not have a supportive fund-
ing policy. That means in some states through public assistance you
would not get a wheelchair—even people with a spinal cord injury.

A wheelchair falls into the category of durable medical equipment (DME) and is often a target of cost controllers in these agencies. They tend to look for the "biggest ticket" items, and try to control spending there. Wheelchairs might seem like just the place to try to save some money, but in fact DME represents only about one percent of total health care spending. But when a cost controller sees a request for a $15,000 power wheelchair, it looks like a good place to control spending, and you might find you will have to fight for approval.

Vocational Rehabilitation and the VA

All states have a program designed to help people with disabilities get back to work after an injury. If you are considered employable—not always an easy status to win if you have a more severe disability—then your state's Vocational Rehabilitation program might invest in education, training, transportation, and, of course, a wheelchair.

Unfortunately, Vocational Rehabilitation funds are also suffering in the '90s, as workers' compensation and disability spending in general have become a target of current politics. In some states, ceilings as low as $16,000 have been imposed on Vocational Rehab cases.

If you are a veteran, you might fare a bit better. The VA is the largest purchaser of wheelchairs in the United States, and the Paralyzed Veterans of America (PVA) is a very substantial and active organization that accomplishes a great deal for its members. They are, at least, a source of considerable information. If you qualify as a veteran, they are a valuable source of assistance for acquiring a chair, as well as for many other needs of people with disabilities.

Alternative funding

If your funding source is refusing to pay for a particular chair or feature, you must decide how long you will fight the good fight. At some point, it is worth more to get on with your life and not have it weighed down by the stress of battling to get coverage. This is a tough choice. You are entitled to what you are entitled to, but you also want good quality of life. At some point it might make sense to take what they give you, and enhance it on your own.

Medicare might not allow you to choose a better chair and simply pay the difference. However, you can enhance the chair they approve—if they won't do it for you—with better positioning systems or other accessories.

The following are some possible sources of funding or finding a chair if you have to "do-it-yourself."

- Your church or other community group might be able to contribute to a purchase or stage a fundraiser on your behalf.

- Many local agencies provide used wheelchairs for people who are not getting proper funding support.

- Your local Independent Living Center might have surplus chairs or parts, or know of someone looking to donate a chair or sell a used one.

- Med-Sell is a newsletter that lists used equipment and accessories. (See the *Resources* section at the end of this book.)

- Some major banks offer special loan programs. For example, San Francisco-based Bank of America offers a longer-term loan with no down payment required if you use it for medical equipment. That can include adaptations to your home or a modified vehicle. The longer term of the loan makes the payments much smaller, helping you handle the cost. Of course, it also means that more interest will accumulate, but if it allows you access to what you need, it might be worth it. Check with major banks in your area to see if they have a similar program.

In all of these cases, of course, you must get proper guidance in identifying what is appropriate for you, including proper cushioning and getting the chair adjusted to your needs.

CHAPTER FOUR

The Selection Process

SELECTING A WHEELCHAIR is a major decision. It is all the more daunting if you are new to the experience. If you've been dreading the moment when it would be necessary, the prospect of having to choose a chair probably feels more like an unpleasant task—or maybe a sentence to prison—than a shopping adventure.

Perhaps you expect a recovery, so you wonder why you should even bother to get a wheelchair at all. No matter how true it is that you might recover, if your physician is recommending a wheelchair, odds are your mobility will be limited for at least a while. There is still a lot of wisdom in getting the right chair. It will optimize your mobility, minimize your fatigue, keep your spirits up by allowing you to be more active, and protect you from hazards that can result from the wrong chair, including some that can impede your recovery. You will want to maintain the best possible health. The right wheels will help you do exactly that.

The professionals who are advising you will talk with you about many issues and options. They will ask you a lot of questions. They may give you catalogs for a variety of chairs that have all kinds of features to choose from. It will likely seem overwhelming. You might think, "Just sell me a wheelchair!"

The best advice is to relax. This is a process that takes time, and it is extremely important not to rush it. You'll have much to learn and many questions to consider. If you find the right people to work with, they will help you identify the chair that will make it possible for you to have the fullest possible life your disability allows. Inform yourself. Trust your advisors, and trust the process.

This chapter will encourage you to begin shopping for your wheelchair when it is time, explains the roles of those who will advise you, and discusses a typical consultation.

When you need one, you need one

Sometimes there is no question about the necessity of obtaining a wheelchair. For instance, if you are coming from a rehab environment where you have been cared for after a sudden disability, you are more likely to realize the need for a chair and look forward to the process of choosing one.

On the other hand, some people—particularly those with a progressive condition—may fall into a gray area. You may be having difficulty walking, but are not sure whether it is time to start using a chair. People with conditions such as multiple sclerosis, some of the muscular dystrophies, or Freidrich's Ataxia, for instance, struggle with when the right moment is to adopt a life on wheels.

Your quite appropriate concern is that you might be surrendering what strength and balance you still have by wheeling instead of walking, but keep in mind that using a wheelchair is not an all or nothing decision. The main priority in your decision should be your safety. If walking puts you at risk of a dangerous fall, you should seriously consider whether maintaining strength is worth that risk. (Remember, exercise can help you keep your strength even if you are using a wheelchair.)

Your emotions at such a time are likely to be complex and confusing. One aspect of your decision whether to start using a chair is probably a discomfort with appearing in public as a chair rider. In the case of this young man with Freidrich's Ataxia, the wheelchair actually improved his sense of public image:

I'm sort of happy about my wheelchair. When I walked with or without support, people—and more importantly, girls—thought I was drunk! They accept me more now that I use wheels.

If you have been doing your best to avoid using a wheelchair, an event that might feel like a surrender or defeat for you, consider that such feelings can interfere with your ability to get the right chair for your needs—the one that will allow you to have the fullest life possible.

Doe Cayting of Wheelchairs of Berkeley observes:

> *People coming into the store (other than those from rehab) are generally unhappy to be here. This is about a permanent lifestyle change. People are horrified. They come in the door thinking, "Sell me a wheelchair, I'll go home with a wheelchair, and that will be the end of it." Then they are appalled at the cost. And the choices are truly overwhelming. However, once people make their decision and accept it, then they get very excited. But getting to that point can be traumatic.*

Do your best to remember that you are not buying a ball and chain, you are buying a device that will extend your mobility. You need only use it when really necessary—you will not be confined to a wheelchair; you will be liberated by it. Often there is a combination of mobility solutions that will protect you while preserving your abilities as much as possible. For example, it might make sense to use a chair when you go out, and then walk at home. You are much better off having a wheelchair around for when you need it. Waiting too long to get a wheelchair can cause a lot more stress.

Who will help you choose your chair?

The prescription for your chair will be written by a physician. You will want to make sure that she is either a rehabilitation specialist (physiatrist) or that she refers you to an occupational or physical therapist who will help ensure that you get the right chair.

Occupational therapist Jody Greenhalgh finds that some people end up with the wrong chair because they relied on their primary physician to specify it.

The primary physician writes a simplistic prescription, and the insurer pays for inadequate equipment. Once that happens, it is very difficult to convince an insurer to pay for a more appropriate wheelchair system.

Physiatrists and rehab therapists understand the medical and physiological issues that affect your wheelchair choices. Some therapists have chosen to make a specialty of consulting on wheelchair selection.

A therapist's knowledge of anatomy and biodynamics is extremely valuable. Your therapist will study your exact disability, and do muscle and range testing. He will determine whether you have the physical ability to push a manual chair, or whether you should drive a power chair. He will identify how to establish a stable posture that will allow you access to your optimal strength as you push, or study your ability to operate the various types of power chair controls. He will test your eye-hand coordination and cognitive skills. He will measure your weight and height, your knee-to-footrest distance, seat depth, back height, and all of the other specific dimensions needed to configure your highly customized set of wheels.

Your therapist is the expert on the specific requirements your physical/medical condition demands from a wheelchair. But keeping up with everything that is available in the wheelchair market is more than most therapists can manage. They can't know it all, so they rely on the wheelchair suppliers who will actually order and sell your wheels.

Your therapist will likely know the best wheelchair dealers to work with, but if you have to find one on your own, the time you spend locating one with knowledge and experience will be well worth it. It's best not to purchase your chair from a general medical supply store, one that sells all sorts of medical equipment. Such a business is not likely to have the kind of expertise you need.

A knowledgeable DME salesperson can make a tremendous difference in ensuring that you get the right wheels. You'll want someone who has a lot of experience seeing many people with different needs, and who has specialized in rehab equipment. A competent salesperson often has more information from users about what worked and what didn't than the therapist does.

If possible, find a salesperson who has experience with insurance and funding. He can help you avoid choosing a product the insurer simply won't pay for, and help you choose appropriate equipment that will be approved.

Doe Cayting of Wheelchairs of Berkeley knows that choosing a first wheelchair is a complex process. The fact that people are being released from rehab earlier than ever before means there are even more factors to consider. Your disability might still be evolving, or you might not know where your permanent residence will be. Cayting's approach takes these variables into consideration:

> We try not to lock you into something, and to foresee as many changes as possible. We have had to learn more about various physical conditions to be able to do a sort of advance planning.

It is important for you to be aware that not every dealer will have this level of expertise. Wheelchair vendors are in a difficult position. They can't carry every product line there is or learn everything there is to know. Some, frankly, don't try very hard. Wheelchair makers and area rehabilitation centers offer chair configuration clinics and seminars that salespeople are encouraged to attend, but not all of them do. Even a conscientious salesperson might be new to the business and still learning.

Bob Hall of New Hall's Wheels, a smaller producer and himself a chair rider, cautions against relying on a dealer who may not be as knowledgeable as one would hope:

> Wheelchair dimensions are often over-prescribed because of lack of knowledge of the dealer. Back heights, in particular, are often too tall and limit movement in the chair. Chairs are often too wide. You can say that you need to make room inside the chair for your winter coat, but if you can't get through the door it isn't doing you

much good. The product actually ends up being more disabling,
whereas the right chair can raise your self-esteem.

You might need to put your dealer to the test, urging him to describe several products.

Another issue to keep in mind is whether the dealer might be influenced by an association with or loyalty to a particular manufacturer, perhaps making a greater profit from one product than another. Ask whether the dealer representative you are working with earns a commission, and try to work with suppliers who can choose from more than one product line.

You may not always have a choice about the dealer with whom you will work. Your funding source might require that you use a particular supplier in order to save money, and such a supplier might not be well informed about the most appropriate product for you. If you believe you need additional consultation in order to get the best chair, assert yourself with your insurance carrier or agency so that you can work with a local source that is better qualified to consult with you.

Even though there are some pitfalls to avoid, there are still many good salespeople with valuable experience who do their best to remain uninfluenced by outside pressures and who truly have your best interest at heart. Karl Ylonen of Care Corporation is committed to making sure that people get the right chair:

> *If someone calls me up and says they want a wheelchair, I want
> to see them. I want to do an evaluation. I want to get a therapist
> involved. It's important to us to involve as many clinical people as
> we can. The most important person in the group is the person
> using the equipment.*

The consultation

A typical consultation will take place at your therapist's office and will include you, your therapist, and a salesperson from your local wheelchair shop. Your therapist will have a list of requirements derived from her work with you. You will have information about your home and workplace, your lifestyle and level of activity, and of course, your personal preferences. (Chapter 5, *Your Role*, discusses your preparation for this consultation.) The salesperson will contribute knowledge about various manufacturers and the products they offer, including necessary accessories, such as cushions, and optional features.

As a team, you will discuss the various factors that will determine the specific features and dimensions of your chair. The therapist and salesperson will guide you through this process, but it is a good idea for you to have some knowledge about the many details that must be taken into consideration. For example, seat height is related to the ground clearance required by footrests. Seat depth is partially dependent on the kind of seat back you choose. As various features are discussed throughout the book, we will alert you to these kinds of interrelationships. The more you know about wheelchair selection, the better you will be able to participate in the process and be the third, crucial participant in this group.

Some decisions need to be made early on, before exact specifications can be written. For example, one of the first things you'll need to think about is the type of cushion you will use. The exact model and size will be needed to determine certain measurements of your chair, such as seat width.

For power chair users, whether the chair will have front-, rear-, or mid-wheel drive is usually one of the first decisions. If you will need a tilt or recline system, this is also considered from the beginning of the process.

Both your therapist and the salesperson want to succeed at getting you the right wheels. The therapist wants to do her job well, and the salesperson wants both you and the therapist to be ongoing customers. They should get you pretty close to the right wheels since they know enough about given disabilities to narrow down the options, but the truth is that only you can determine what is optimal for you. Be assertive about your preferences and priorities at the same time as you make the most of learning from their expertise.

You should be given the chance to try out a close configuration of the chair you will eventually purchase. The supplier should have chairs on hand that can be adjusted fairly closely to your needs, and may even allow you to take it out and live with it for a few days. Some manufacturers will actually ship a chair to the supplier specifically for you to try out.

One rider describes his experience with the selection process:

> I spent two days with a team in making my decision. The team included a physical therapist and an occupational therapist. The physical therapist spent time assessing my strengths and weaknesses. We then decided on seating requirements before addressing the actual chair selection. We spent a lot of time discussing my lifestyle and exactly how and where the chair was to be used.
>
> Once the medical needs were identified and physical measurements were taken, the last thing was to determine the exact model of chair. We were able to narrow it down to five, which I was able to try out for a few hours each. The trial included maneuvering in a simulation of the work area I use and then spending an hour or so outside on a variety of terrains. We also tried them in my van to see how they fit and the method of transfer I would need to use to get in the driver's seat.
>
> Luckily, I knew enough to demand this sort of evaluation and knew where to go to get competent professional help.

Ordering your chair

From your initial consultation to the actual ordering of your chair typically takes two to three months. (If it's not your first chair, it may take less time.) This includes taking time to try out one or more models. A more complex chair may take longer. If you encounter resistance from your insurer, that could also add time to the process.

Once you have decided on the model of chair that is best for you, the dealer—using information from you and your therapist—will fill out a specification sheet with the exact details for every aspect of your chair. Ask to see a copy of this list. If you have questions or concerns about anything, ask. Make sure it is complete and correct; if something is inadvertently omitted (such as clothing guards) or wrong (such as color), you'll end up with a chair that isn't what you wanted. Even if the problem can be fixed, you'll probably have to pay for it. Your therapist will sign off on this list, and it will then go to your physician, who will write a prescription for it.

The prescription and specification list will be sent to your insurance company or funding agency for approval. Once approved, the dealer will order your chair from the manufacturer. (For steps to take if your insurer denies the chair your doctor prescribes, see Chapter 3, *Who Pays for Your Chair?*) If your chair is not covered by insurance and you are paying for it yourself, a down payment of 50 percent at the time the order is placed is typical.

Your dealer should give you an accurate delivery date so you can plan accordingly.

CHAPTER FIVE

Your Role

IT IS VERY IMPORTANT to get as close as you can to the optimal chair for you when you make your selection. You could wait years before your financial source is willing to buy another. Funders often won't pay even for minor changes like different tires or additional accessories like a knapsack or crutch holder once you accept delivery of your chair.

No matter how skilled and knowledgeable your therapist and salesperson are, you are the expert on you. Since you are the person who will have to live with your wheelchair, it is in your best interest to take an active role in its selection, to learn as much as you can, and to take your time before making the final choice.

This chapter will help you be an effective member of your selection team, cooperating to arrive at the best solution. It will tell you how doing your own research, sharing thorough information about relevant issues in your life, and keeping an open mind will help ensure that you get the chair that will work best for you.

Do some research

Chances are you know other chair users, possibly from your rehab experience, support groups, participation in athletics, or your local independent living center. Chair users tend to be very opinionated about their choices. Remember that every person is different. You can learn much from what others say, but what works best for them might not work for you.

My experience with purchasing the best chair for me came primarily from my own research, which included talking with other wheelchair users. I got a couple of names from the retailer, but the best information I got was from the Internet.

Check the track record of all chairs under consideration. There could be defects in the manufacture of some chairs, as with any consumer product. The U.S. Food and Drug Administration (FDA) keeps track of voluntary recalls by wheelchair manufacturers, although not all manufacturers are entirely open about such problems. While major flaws are uncommon, you can contact the FDA for this information. Newer manufacturers should not be suspect just because they are less experienced, but there is always some risk of unforeseen problems that simply may not have appeared yet. Seek out users of a given product and speak with them about its performance and quality before selecting your wheels.

You might also want to do some research to understand how wheelchairs are tested, and what standards for conformity exist. In 1982, standard procedures for testing and comparing wheelchairs were established by the American National Standards Institute (ANSI) and the Rehabilitation Engineering and Assistive Technology Society of North America (RESNA). Supported by the Paralyzed Veterans of America and the U.S. Department of Veterans Affairs, the Wheelchair Standards Committee did an exhaustive study of wheelchairs and produced the *ANSI/RESNA Guide to Wheelchair Selection*.

The ANSI/RESNA tests and standards make it possible to compare one chair to another. For instance, in the past it was not clear whether seat width was measured from inside or outside the armrests. Some tests are performed with weighted dummies so that dimensions and performance will mimic what happens when you are actually using your chair, since its dimensions change when it is bearing weight. Other tests include finding the limits of tipping angles, fire resistance, and even the ability to withstand being dropped.

ANSI/RESNA testing is not legally mandatory for manufacturers, but since the VA requires test results for all chairs they purchase, most chair manufacturers are using these uniform test procedures.

Actual testing is often performed under contract by groups such as the University of Pittsburgh Department of Rehabilitation Science and Technology, which works with several major manufacturers. Test results are available to the public, so you can know you are comparing apples to apples. However, manufacturers do not typically include the results in their standard consumer literature. It is usually necessary to call them and request results for the products you are interested in. You can also purchase the booklet that details the tests and criteria from the PVA, listed in the *Resources* section at the end of this book.

Learn as much as possible about chairs and what is available on the market. (Chapter 2, *Large Versus Small Manufacturers*, discusses the advantages and drawbacks of choosing a product from a big name producer or from a smaller company.) You can request product information from all companies that appear to have something you think might work for you. Wheelchair manufacturers not only have catalogs and brochures available, but they can provide a specific checklist for every model that includes all available options.

Dr. Michael Boninger, of the University of Pittsburgh, observes:

> This is a crazy industry. It is hard to be a vendor. They might not show you an option that could be best for you because they don't carry it or don't know about it. You can only benefit from learning more on your own.

If you have a good idea of your options before you meet with your therapist and salesperson to actually make a decision, you'll be in a better position to evaluate their recommendations. Jeff Ewing of Falcon Rehabilitation, makers of a power wheelchair and recline systems, agrees:

> I've sat in on a lot of wheelchair clinics, and everything is presented so fast that it's overwhelming. The users hear it all at once and can't understand exactly what's going on. They'll end up getting stuck with something that isn't what they need. It'll be four or five years before they're eligible to get another one, especially if it's a power chair, which funding sources will not easily replace.

Don't hesitate to ask as many questions of the people on your team as it takes for you to have a clear understanding of your choices. Be patient, and insist that they be patient with you. Don't allow yourself to be rushed to a decision before you feel confident that you have enough information to make the right one.

Be prepared for your consultation

Your wheelchair supplier will need to know many things about where you live and work. It is not uncommon for an occupational or physical therapist to visit you and make notes about your living space, but you will want to take an active part in making sure your chair will optimize—not limit—your mobility and comfort at home and work. Investigate your home and workplace, and then arrive at your therapist appointment or the wheelchair store equipped with answers to questions such as these:

- How wide are your doors—main entry, kitchen, bedrooms, bathrooms, etc.?

- Are there tight angles to negotiate, such as a hallway that turns sharply at the bedroom door?

- How large is the bathroom? Will it be possible to wheel your chair alongside the bathtub, or must you face it directly? Is the door smaller than the others in your house? Will you be able to close the door once inside with your wheelchair?

- What is the knee clearance of tables and desks?

- How high are cabinets and shelves that you might need to reach?

- Is the terrain around your home paved? If not, what kind of surface is it? Is it level?

- What are the surfaces where you will do most of your wheeling? Carpet, tile, concrete, packed soil?

You must also consider the vehicles you use:

- If you drive, do you have a car or a van? Two or four doors?

- What is the size of the trunk in the family car?

- What kind of public transportation might you use?

Failure to consider any one of these points can mean having to live with a constant irritant or insurmountable obstacle, and facing the stress of unnecessary restriction of your mobility every day—just because you got the wrong chair. You might even be risking your safety if, for instance, you are forced to make a long transfer to the bath or shower because you chose those fixed footrests, which prevent you from getting close enough.

Getting the right chair can also save you from having to make potentially expensive home modifications.

It was many years before we could make my home wheelchair accessible. If I had known that there were power wheelchairs out there that could raise a seated person 6 to 8 inches or that had a turning radius of 19.5 inches, my life would have been so much more comfortable. And it wouldn't have cost quite so much for the home modifications.

You will also want to share important information about your lifestyle and the kinds of activities you plan to participate in. If you like to be on the go—visiting friends, attending entertainment and sporting events, taking classes—or travel a lot either for pleasure or business, you might need a different chair than if you prefer a more quiet life and enjoy being home most of the time. Information about your preferences is critical. Along with the previous lists, make one that includes:

- Hobbies and activities for which your chair will be a consideration.

- Relevant information about any "homes away from home." If you like to hang out at your best friend's place, you want to make sure you can fit through those doors, too.

- The importance of the appearance of your chair to you. Do you see yourself in something sporty? Eye-catching? Or do looks not matter much to you?

- Your usual level of physical activity, including exercise.

Your lifestyle and personal preferences for comfort are important. Without your input, your team might not fully understand your needs. The more information about yourself that you can give to the therapist and salesperson, the better they can help you identify the chair that will work best for you.

Although my rehab folks were wonderful, my first two chairs did not suit my lifestyle. There were places I might have been able to go, people I might have been able to see, and events I could have participated in if I had had the right chair from the beginning.

Keep an open mind

Despite the variety of wheelchairs on the market, and the many options available, you may not be able to find every feature and detail you would ideally like in one chair. As with other purchases, such as a car or home, some compromises and trade-offs are usually necessary. As you work your way through the selection process, try to think about the big picture and how you will use your chair over time. Establish priorities, learn from the experience of others, and value the advice of experts.

You'll also want to weigh carefully the benefits and drawbacks of each option. It's unwise to be so fixed on a certain choice that you deny yourself the chance to gain a complete perspective. Doe Cayting of Wheelchairs of Berkeley describes such a situation:

Some people are adamant that they don't want to have to swing away the footrest—ever! You have to respect their input, but the reality for one person was that instead of going to live in an apartment, he went to a family member's house where he cannot get close enough to the bathtub in a rigid chair with fixed footrests. So this feature that he was absolutely sure about has become an absolute nightmare.

It is common for people to be drawn to the appearance of a chair, but it is dangerous to be overly influenced by the look of a chair to the possible exclusion of other, more important issues. That really cool-looking rigid-frame chair might not fit into the trunk of your family car.

Cayting has seen people become too attached to the appearance of the chair, in lieu of other features more important to their mobility:

> You have to think about whether aesthetics is the most important thing for you, because the right chair is always a question of compromise. There isn't an exact right or wrong. But if you want something that looks a certain way, and I know it is not appropriate, it is my responsibility as a supplier to say no.

Fortunately, there are lots of good-looking chairs that fit many needs. Compared to the institutional-style chair that everyone had to use until the 1980s, whatever you choose will be better looking and more to your liking than in "the old days."

Buying from a catalog

You need the guidance and advice of your therapist and wheelchair dealer when you purchase your first chair. When you need an additional chair or need to replace a chair, the process will be more familiar. Once you become experienced enough, you might even bypass the experts, and take advantage of discount mail order houses that deal in top-line models. Discount houses offer lower prices because they are not paying a sales staff to provide you hours of consultation. But you will have to do lots of your own research, and do it well. You are also unlikely to get a chance to try out a chair before buying.

Direct catalog suppliers realize their customers are knowledgeable, often simply replacing the exact chair they were already using. Typically, these customers only need to hear about new features or updated designs they should consider, but they are well versed in dimensions. Such customers usually read the disability magazines, so have kept up on changes in wheelchair design.

However, it's important to know your limits when it comes to do-it-yourself wheelchair selection. Catalog suppliers should make an effort to ensure that you are getting what you need. If they sense that you are asking for the wrong chair, they should urge you to get a local assessment, and you should listen to that advice.

Power chair users need to be particularly cautious about purchasing a new chair without benefit of professional advice. Karl Ylonen of Care Corporation explains his view:

> For power chairs, a physical assessment should be done every time. Period. I feel pretty strongly about that. You're talking about an expensive piece of equipment. Generally people who are using power have more disadvantages physically than someone in a manual chair. It's important to make sure power chair users are getting what they need.

Before you decide to buy a chair through a direct catalog, remember that you will forgo some of the benefits of an ongoing relationship with a local dealer, such as preventive maintenance services at no charge.

Have your new chair properly adjusted

When your chair arrives at the dealer from the factory, you will need to have the store adjust it specifically to your needs. Plan on taking the time to have them fine-tune it for you, and don't hesitate to ask them to continue to make changes until it is right. Dr. Boninger, of the University of Pittsburgh, finds that factory settings are not particularly optimal overall. For example, he makes this observation about manual chairs:

> The factory tends to put the wheels far back for stability, but this can force excessive range of motion as you reach back, and limit the amount of stroke you can make on the wheel.

Axle position is only one of the many details of chair configuration that have a significant impact on the efficient, comfortable, and safe use of your chair. Remember that a wheelchair is really a complex web of interrelationships. Changing the axle position or caster height affects seat and back angles, and the relationship of your arms to the wheels. Placement of a joystick affects overall posture. And so on.

Some riders learn—by observing and asking questions of a qualified technician—how to expertly adjust their own chairs, but you should not attempt to adjust your chair until you are confident in your knowledge and are certain that you have the right tools to protect the chair from scratches and to avoid stripping the heads of screws or bolts. More than one wheelchair salesperson can tell a story of a customer who called complaining that their chair was wrong or damaged, only to discover that they had made inappropriate adjustments or used the wrong tools.

Some things just need time to settle in. A new folding wheelchair will be a little harder to open and close, but will loosen up with use. New tires with fresh tread will wear on your hands more at first. But achieving and maintaining optimal adjustment is very important, and it is your responsibility to make it happen.

CHAPTER SIX

The Basic Choice: Manual or Power

THE FIRST DECISION TO BE MADE when choosing your wheelchair is whether it will be a manual or power chair. Are you going to push or drive? Or both?

Typical manual chair riders include those with lower spinal cord injuries, neuromuscular conditions that affect only the lower extremities, many post-polio individuals, and amputees. These riders most likely have the upper-body balance, arm strength, and dexterity to propel themselves in a manual "push" chair.

High-level quadriplegic riders and those without sufficient arm strength or coordination clearly need a power chair.

Those who fall into either of the above populations don't need to decide whether a manual or power chair is best—their choice is obvious. For others, the choice is not so simple and, in fact, it sometimes takes both kinds of chairs to reach the optimal solution.

Two chairs are actually a good idea for everyone—manual and power chair riders alike will want to have a backup manual chair for use in case their main chair is out of commission for a few days. A backup chair doesn't have to be as complete or as customized as one you purchase for daily use. If you aren't able to get your own backup chair, find out if your dealer has loaners available for those times when your chair needs servicing.

This chapter will explore some of the factors to consider if you're unsure whether a power or manual chair will serve you best.

Advantages of manual wheelchairs

Manual chairs have a number of advantages over power chairs, and most people prefer to use a manual chair if at all possible. Consider the following list of "pros," but also be honest with yourself about your strength and energy—you'll need plenty of both to operate a manual chair.

- Manual chairs are lightweight, and getting lighter all the time, thanks to modern metal alloys and composite materials. Lightweight chairs require less strength and energy to push than their predecessors.

- Manual chairs have unlimited range, since they are not tied to the charge capacity of a battery.

- Manual chairs cost less to purchase than power chairs. Maintenance costs are also lower thanks to fewer working parts and not needing to replace depleted batteries.

- Manual chairs, since they are less bulky, are more discreet than power chairs, and, with no motor noise, they are quieter—assuming the manual chair is well maintained.

- Manual chairs are easier to maneuver for slight rotations or small movements, although the newer controls for power chairs are excellent.

- Manual chairs travel more easily than power chairs, whether on an airplane or in the backseat or trunk of a car. Depending on options, a manual chair can be stored more easily when broken down to its component parts. Swingaway footrests can be removed, as can the wheels by means of the now-common quick-release axles.

- Manual chairs can extend mobility. For those with the strength and agility to master the art of the "wheelie," many curbs and single steps no longer represent an obstacle in a manual chair, as you can safely "jump" a curb or step, going either up or down.

Advantages of power wheelchairs

Some riders are finding that they do better in a power chair as they age. Chronic shoulder pain from overuse or weakness from an illness might make it necessary. Some of the reasons you might opt for a power chair are:

- A power chair preserves your energy, allowing you to go whatever distance necessary without exhausting yourself for work or pleasure activities.

- A power chair allows you to handle uphill slopes that would be an unnecessary overexertion or perhaps beyond your ability to climb with a manual chair.

- A power chair frees you from the need for assistance from another when going a considerable distance or on a steep surface.

- A power chair leaves one arm free to stabilize an object you might carry in your lap—such as a bag of groceries or books—while operating a joystick control.

- A power chair can include powered tilt or recline features, which aid in pressure-sore prevention, respiration, and comfort for quadriplegic riders.

Weigh your options

Choosing a power chair can be a tough decision. There are mobility restrictions that come along with use of a power chair. Power chairs are limited by battery life, are too heavy to be carried up a stairway, and don't jump curbs easily, if at all. They make more noise and are less able to make fine maneuvers. Pushing a manual chair keeps the upper body in shape, to a degree, so using a power chair can be an invitation to lose strength.

Some people resist choosing a power chair because it makes them feel "too disabled." But it's important to ask yourself how much of your daily energy you are willing to invest in pushing a manual chair. If you have marginal upper-body strength, you can exhaust yourself just getting where you're going. Perhaps you are attending a college that is on a sloping site or live in a hilly town. Consider whether you prefer to trade having more energy in the day against your public image as a power chair rider. Lack of energy from pushing a manual chair around might even make a difference in your ability to hold a job.

Finally, think about how the effort needed to operate a manual chair will affect your health in the long run. Many manual chair riders with twenty or so years of pushing behind them find that their shoulders begin to give out. You are better off using a manual chair if you can, but not at the expense of your long-term health.

Using a combination of manual and power chairs

Many low-level quadriplegic people have sufficient arm strength to push a chair, perhaps aided by handrims with knobs, which are easier to grasp than rims alone. Some of these riders use a manual chair at all times, while others switch between manual and power chairs, depending on distance, surface, and whether they might need to be lifted up stairs, load the chair into a car, etc. You might use a power chair to go to and from work, but use a manual chair at home and at the office. A blend of the two types can be the ideal strategy for your mobility. It is an approach that does not waste your energy or overuse your body.

There have been some interesting efforts at a "best of both worlds" solution. The Roll-Aid is a motorized unit that attaches to a manual, folding wheelchair. You roll over it until the steering/control arm is between your legs, and the Roll-Aid will attach itself to your chair, allowing you to drive it like a scooter, steering with two hands rather than using a single joystick, as with most power chairs.

The Quickie P200 model has revolutionized power chairs in a variety of ways. One of its unique characteristics is that the basic chair unit can be lifted off the motor module, and then manual wheels can be attached.

Scooters—an option for some

So far we have talked about choosing either a manual or power wheelchair, or using some combination of both. Although wheelchairs are the focus of this book, a scooter is another option that deserves mention. A scooter can increase mobility for those who need assistance only occasionally, or who can use a manual chair most of the time. Some people find scooters to be more socially acceptable than a wheelchair.

Scooters have the advantage of being motorized, while also being generally less costly than a power chair. For those with good arm strength and upper-body balance, a scooter might be a good

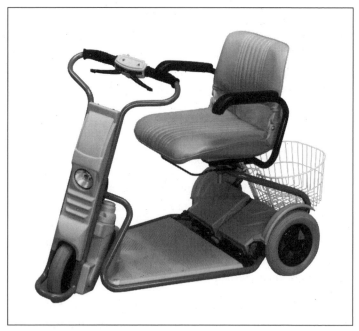

Figure 1. A lightweight, three-wheeled scooter

solution. Figure 1, "A lightweight, three-wheeled scooter," is an example of a typical scooter.

A scooter is often used by people who are able to walk to some degree, but are challenged by distances and slopes. Scooters are popular with elderly users and people with progressive conditions such as multiple sclerosis, muscular dystrophy, or amyotrophic lateral sclerosis when their walking is limited.

Even if you are unable to stand, a scooter may still have a role to play in your mobility.

> As a manual chair user, I own a scooter to climb some streets in my neighborhood in San Francisco. I also use it to go greater distances since I became concerned about the effect on my arms and shoulders from pushing a manual chair those distances. I find it useful for shopping, because rather than place merchandise in my lap while I wheel, I can carry it between my feet. You may also opt for a wire basket which hangs on the steering arm in front of you.

Given the fact that you steer a scooter—rather than control its direction with a joystick—you need sufficient arm strength to drive one, as well as the use of your thumbs to press the controls.

Most scooters are equipped with a captain's chair that has vinyl- or cloth-covered foam upholstery. Traditionally, the cushioning has not been designed for the kinds of advanced pressure relief that many people with disabilities require. Those with special cushioning needs have had to find a scooter with an adaptive seating option that accepts pressure-relief products. Happily, scooters are getting more attention from designers, and more models of this type are beginning to appear.

It is unusual for someone to spend the whole day in a scooter, the way full-time chair riders do with a wheelchair. Compared to a power wheelchair, a scooter is set apart by a variety of features:

- A tiller centered in front of the body steers a single front wheel. This arm can be tilted forward or backward and locked at any desired position.

- Thumb levers are used to drive the scooter, usually pressing with the right thumb to go forward, the left to reverse.

- The seat, mounted on a stem, can rotate to the sides and is held in place by a lock/release mechanism.

- Rather than footrests, the scooter is designed with a base platform that carries the seat and batteries and supports your feet.

Most scooters have three wheels, but some have four. Three-wheeled scooters are less stable and may tip over when taking a corner too fast, or when turning on a surface with a sideways slope, like a sidewalk. Four-wheeled scooters are more difficult to steer and so require more strength and dexterity to drive.

Scooters are usually equipped with automatic braking, so they do not coast. You must apply the controls for all movement. A knob to set the maximum speed is usually included with the controls. Scooter controls are not as sophisticated as the new breed of power wheelchairs, which include programming for acceleration and braking, among other advanced features. This means that, with a scooter, you must press and release the controls gently to modulate how quickly you start and slow down. Some scooter controls have a built-in delay to prevent sudden starts, but some users find it irritating to have to wait the extra moments to start each time they press the control. Control systems are another feature that are likely to be improved by increased interest in scooters on the part of manufacturers.

The better scooter designs provide you with subtle controls that allow you to make small and slow movements. You need not fear that you will have trouble controlling a scooter if you have sufficient upper-body control. However, you must take care not to press a drive lever accidentally by catching your jacket on it, for instance. To prevent accidental movement, most scooters are key operated so that you can turn them off while you are at a standstill. A gear release will allow you to disengage the drive mechanism if you need to push the scooter manually.

Since there is a steering arm in front of you, scooters don't work very well at tables and desks. You can't just wheel up to them, but instead have to pull alongside, rotate the seat, and then pull the table toward your body. When you are turned to the side, there is no longer support for your feet. Practical issues like these are why a scooter is best for a neighborhood shopping trip, exploring a nature trail, or taking an accessible bus ride to the city for an appointment, but not so ideal for everyday use, particularly at work, unless you are able to stand and get into another chair.

Scooters can be broken down into component parts to be stowed in a car trunk, making them useful for outings with family and friends. The process takes a bit of strength and dexterity, but is very manageable with a couple of able-bodied helpers. Newer designs are getting lighter and easier to break down and transport.

Depending on the amount of power you need, such as to climb ramps or moderate slopes, choose a scooter with either one or two batteries. A charger should also be included.

CHAPTER SEVEN

Manual Chair Decisions

YOU HAVE DETERMINED THAT YOU NEED a manual wheelchair. As you've learned, there are many more decisions to make before you ride away in your ideal wheels. Some decisions, such as what type of cushion to choose, or whether to choose solid rubber or pneumatic tires, are not unique to manual chair riders. Chapters 9 through 14 discuss features common to both manual and power chairs.

However, as someone who will be manually pushing a chair, you have some specific choices to make that will affect the ease with which you maneuver your wheels. This chapter offers considerations for deciding between a rigid frame or a folding frame, points out the importance of chair weight as well as wheel size and angle, and discusses handrims and wheel locks.

Rigid or folding?

It used to be that most manual wheelchairs folded. Now there are rigid designs that offer a number of advantages over folding chairs. Rigid chairs have become widely popular among riders because they are easy to push, responsive, light, strong, and have a streamlined appearance. However, rigid chairs can be bulky for transporting in a car and do not neatly fold up when they need to be out of the way. They can be somewhat unstable when moving over uneven terrain. Figure 2, "A lightweight, rigid-frame manual wheelchair," shows a typical rigid chair.

There are a few important reasons why some riders still prefer folding chairs. Their ability to fold into a compact unit offers convenience. For example, folding chairs are likely to fit in most vehicles. The flexible frame of folding chairs enables them to stay stable over bumpy surfaces. But folding chairs take more energy to push than rigid chairs and lack the other attractive qualities of the rigid design. Figure 3, "A lightweight, folding manual wheelchair," shows a typical folding chair.

An engineer will tell you that when you push a folding wheelchair, some energy is lost in the flexibility of the frame. Not all of the work of your push translates into forward motion. The loss of energy in a flexible frame led chair designers to come up with the rigid-frame chair. Freed of the mechanism for folding, a rigid chair has fewer parts and is therefore much lighter. With fewer moving components, the frame has more strength. More of the energy of your push translates into motion. The rigid chair design also allows for the angle of the seat frame to be adjustable, impossible with a folding chair. The cross-frame design of the folding chair is not needed with a rigid chair, streamlining the rigid chair's appearance. The rigid-frame design has come to be a *de facto* standard for those who want to reduce the visual emphasis on their disability.

Rigid-frame chairs are so responsive that just minor movements of your body can be enough to adjust direction—a technique riders can use to make some of the fine adjustments necessary as they wheel. Some people find rigid chairs a little oversensitive, but many swear by them and will never go back to a folding design. According to Doe Cayting of Wheelchairs of Berkeley:

> We like rigid frames because in a folding chair forty percent of your energy is wasted by the mechanism of the frame. Greater efficiency means you won't tire as easily, and you won't have to worry so much about overuse syndrome.

Some find a rigid chair necessary because of its more rugged construction:

> I prefer my rigid-frame chair. I may be inconvenienced at times when I can't get close to a table, but this is rare since my chair is quite short and the ends of my toes sit directly below my knees. The durability of a rigid frame is essential, as I am quite hard on

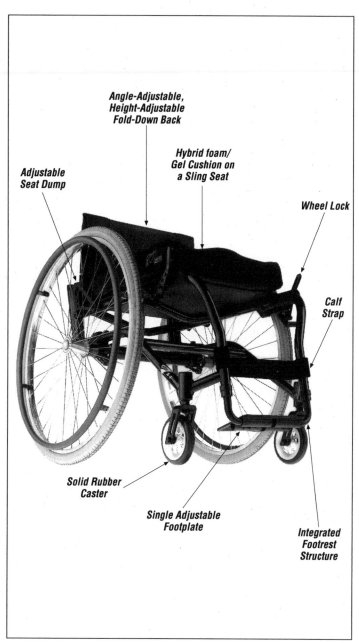

Figure 2. A lightweight, rigid-frame manual wheelchair

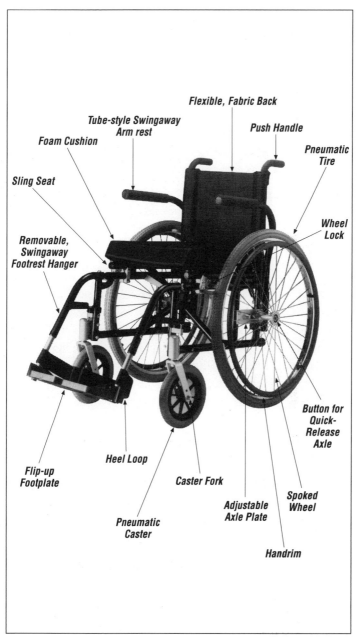

Figure 3. A lightweight, folding manual wheelchair

my equipment and it must endure Ottawa winters. It has few moving parts to loosen, collect dirt, and break. The chair requires less maintenance.

Rigid chairs are generally considered less convenient to carry in vehicles (unless you drive a lift- or ramp-equipped van), but whether you find it easier to load a folding or rigid chair into your car depends on the size and style of your vehicle, your upper-body strength, the length of your arms, and other factors. One rider votes for the rigid chair as easier to load:

As a recent purchaser of a fixed frame, I consider it superior to the folding ones. I can get it into the backseat by putting it over the passenger seat back, but it is easier just to leave it in the passenger seat. I never did find a way to enter on the driver's side with my folding chair.

To load a rigid chair into a car, it is necessary to remove the wheels (easily accomplished with quick-release axles) and fold the back of the chair down against the seat. The remaining rigid frame without the wheels can be somewhat bulky, requiring sufficient upper-body strength and balance to pull the frame into the car. Some drivers enter from the passenger side, pulling the frame in after them, others recline back in the driver's seat and pull the frame over their body to place it on the passenger seat. Keep in mind that if you need to put your chair in the trunk, a rigid chair might not allow the trunks of some cars to close.

Some riders prefer a folding chair as their best overall solution for a daily street chair because of its ability to fold into a more compact unit:

Even though I tried a rigid-frame chair, and sure, it was easier to wheel and looked better, I found it much harder to put in my two-door car. It wouldn't fit in the trunk either. I also feel strongly about keeping my chair with me in theaters, and a rigid chair would block the aisles, so I would have to let them take it away

during the show. I have enough upper-body strength and balance
to push a folding chair without tiring myself, so for these and other
reasons, a folding design is still the style of choice for my needs.

You will want to consider what kind of terrain you will be traveling over. On uneven surfaces, all four wheels of a folding chair are better able to remain in contact with the surface because of its flexible frame. The flexible frame also absorbs small bumps and vibrations in your ride. Rigid frames are best for hard, reasonably level surfaces. On uneven terrain, a rigid chair will give you a harder ride, and might have one or more wheels lift off the ground, preventing you from being able to wheel. This loss of control can be dangerous.

One way to compensate for the limited ability of a rigid chair to provide a smooth ride is to take advantage of the recent development of rigid frames that have shock absorbers—usually for the main wheels, but they can also be found for casters. The shock absorbers help soften the ride of the rigid frame and keep all four wheels in contact with the ground more of the time, but you don't sacrifice as much of your work in pushing as you would with a folding frame.

Playing sports

Serious sports enthusiasts use highly specialized chairs, such as those designed for tennis, basketball, rugby, or racing, and have another chair—perhaps folding—for everyday use. The focus of this book is on helping you choose your daily chair, so the various possibilities for sport chairs is beyond its scope. (At the back of the book, the *Resources* section include several manufacturers that specialize in sport chairs.)

Not everyone has the funds for two wheelchairs, however, and some just want to enjoy athletic activities at a casual level without having to make a big investment. Some sports organizations have helped with the problem by having sport chairs available at their events. Some basketball teams try to raise funds to purchase chairs that can be dedicated to sports use.

If you want to find a daily chair that can also hold up and function properly during sports, you'll need to put some extra thought into it.

For example, a daily chair needs to be as narrow as possible to make sure you can get through tight aisles in some stores and navigate your home easily. You might need the additional support of a taller back since you will sit for more hours without moving. You might need push handles, particularly if you have friends whose homes you visit by getting a lift up steps. A folding chair might be necessary for travel or if you drive a two-door car. If you do business, it might be important to keep the chair more conservative looking. You might prefer larger pneumatic tires for a softer ride on the street.

For sporting activities, the maneuverability and quickness of a rigid chair is preferable. You need more camber on the wheels for stability, and a lower back without handles to free your upper body to move in as wide a range as possible. Small—but hard—casters give you more agility. You might also prefer a jazzy color scheme.

So what options are there to address these conflicting needs? To begin with, you could have two sets of casters, or another set of main wheels with thin profile tires, made of a lighter material. Another set of back canes without push handles could be changed without too much trouble. In other words, by purchasing a few extra parts, you can reconfigure your street chair for sports—to a degree.

A couple of manufacturers are trying to take on this issue. The Invacare Action A-4 has optional quick-release mechanisms for changing both wheel camber and front casters. The seat angle can be changed without much difficulty.

The Quickie TNT (Takes No Tools) was introduced in 1998 to offer a chair that can be easily adjusted on the fly. Camber, axle position, caster height, seat angle, backrest height and angle, and wheel lock positions can all be changed quickly with no tools. It can be configured with many of the other options typical of a chair—like push handles and sideguards—but cannot use pneumatic casters because of its tight footrest hanger angle.

Clearly the wheelchair industry is taking note that people with disabilities have lifestyles as varied as the general population and increasingly need more flexibility in what one set of wheels will do. Chances are the future will see this category of wheelchair continue to evolve.

Comparison of Rigid and Folding Manual Wheelchairs

Chair type	Advantages	Disadvantages
Rigid	Fewer parts. Lighter. Stronger. Easier to push. Responsive. Streamlined appearance. Adjustable seat frame angle. More appropriate for athletic activities.	May not fit in vehicle or may be difficult to load. Can't be made as compact, to put out of the way when not in use. Less control on uneven surfaces. Rougher ride (may be helped by shock absorbers).
Folding	Convenient. Fits in most vehicles. Stable over bumpy surfaces. Absorbs vibrations.	Requires more energy to push. More parts mean more servicing. Somewhat heavier. Can't adjust seat frame angle. Less streamlined appearance.

Chair weight

The heavier your manual chair, the more energy you will use to push it. A heavier chair is also more difficult for anyone assisting you, making it harder to push you a long distance, carry you up a stairway, or store your chair when you're not in it. Will your grandmother need to lift the chair into the trunk of a car?

Steel chair frames are the heaviest, but are now less common. The majority of chairs use an aluminum alloy, which is light in weight, but strong. Titanium is an extremely light metal that is also very strong, but it is expensive. Titanium is used primarily for racing chairs, but you will find it used for certain components such as wheel rims or axle shafts. Spoked wheels are lighter than molded wheels, but require more maintenance. Air-filled tires are less heavy than solid tires.

Total weight is also affected by the type of cushion you use, gel-filled cushions being the heaviest, and urethane and foam cushions the lightest. As you make the many choices necessary to define the best chair for you, you will want to consider chair weight versus the advantages of some features that will make it heavier.

An important safety issue with a light chair is that it has a longer braking distance. You'll want to remember this while getting used to your wheels.

> When I made the transition from the hospital-style aluminum chair to a modern lightweight, I discovered that I had less traction against the pavement, and so had to allow for a greater distance to slow down. It only took one close call to learn that lesson!

Size and type of wheels

Your optimal reach for pushing will be determined in part by the diameter of the wheels. Manual chairs typically use 24-inch wheels, but wheels are available as small as 20 inches and as large as 26 inches. If you must begin a push with your arms already extended because the wheels are small or you are sitting too high, you will have very little remaining force. If you begin the push with your elbows very bent and your shoulders raised because the wheels are large or you are sitting too low, you will be overstraining your arms and shoulders to get the chair to start moving.

Wheel diameter must work in conjunction with seat height. The sequence of events leading to the decision for wheel diameter goes something like this: first you must ensure proper ground clearance for your footrests based on your leg length. Then you can determine minimum seat height, and from seat height you can determine seat angle. A seat lower at the back will bring your arms closer to the wheels and rims. Only after you know how high and at what angle your seat will be can you determine your appropriate wheel size. If you want to use larger wheels, which can be easier to push, you might choose a seat height that is greater than the minimum.

You will also have a choice of what type of wheels you want. One of the innovations of the Quickie wheelchair was the use of molded wheels. Molded wheels can endure more impact than the old-fashioned spoked wheels, which have a way of getting knocked out of adjustment.

After years of bouncing up and down curbs in my old Everest & Jennings chair—much heavier than my present Quickie—my wheels were so knocked out of shape that they looked absolutely wavy if you watched from behind.

The molded wheel design contributed much to breaking the hospital stereotype of previous chairs. Molded wheels continue to be available. However, spoked wheels have returned to favor with a new design in which the spokes do not cross over each other at the hub. This new spoke design is good looking and helps the spokes maintain their tension.

Placement and angle of wheels

Two important decisions for chair stability and optimal wheeling efficiency are where the wheel axle will be in relation to the back of the chair, and the amount of angle, or camber, on the wheels.

With most modern manual chairs, you can adjust the axle position forward or backward in relation to the back of the chair. This is the point of pivot, where your weight is applied to the chair. When the wheel is moved forward on the axle, more of the chair weight is behind the axle, so it will tip more easily, lifting the front casters off the ground. At the least you want to be able to slightly lift the casters with a bit of extra push to soften your ride over bumps in the sidewalk, for instance. At most, you might use the technique of doing wheelies to go up and down curbs. The axle position will control how efficiently you can perform these maneuvers without putting yourself at risk of falling backward in your chair. When you get a new chair, you might begin with a more stable rearward position, and then move the axle forward as you gain more experience driving.

Correct wheel position is also determined by your weight, and how your weight is proportioned. For example, taller people have longer legs, and so have more body weight forward in the chair. More weight forward in the chair allows for a more forward wheel position without risk of falling. If you wear heavy shoes or boots, you might take that into account by moving the wheels forward. Amputees have much less forward body weight, so must use a rearward wheel position. They might even require a chair frame that allows the axle to be placed behind the vertical line of the chair back.

If the wheels are too far back, they can be hard to reach for pushing, forcing you to pull your arms farther back. Forward tipping also becomes a risk factor. When the wheels are farther back, your chair will want to roll toward the street on sidewalks, which are always sloped toward the street for water drainage. You will have to push harder on the downhill wheel to compensate for gravity pulling the front end sideways.

Another decision is the amount of camber you want on your wheels. Camber is the angle of the wheels toward your body as they rise from the floor (see Figure 4, "A specialized sport chair with cambered wheels"). Some rigid-frame chairs are available in various fixed camber angles, where the axle housing is welded in place at the given angle. Most chairs use an adjustable plate that holds the axle and allows the camber to be changed.

The greater the camber, the wider the wheelbase, and therefore the greater the lateral stability of the chair as you turn corners or lean over. Athletic chairs used for racing, tennis, rugby, and so on have severe camber angles. Those things really move fast! The camber is necessary to keep them—and the riders—upright. In a day-to-day chair you want less camber because the added width at the floor makes it difficult to pass through narrow spaces. It is extremely common in a chair rider's life that a matter of a quarter of an inch can make the difference in getting where you need to go.

A different kind of wheel angle—one which you want to avoid—is "toe-in" or "toe-out." If your wheels were to roll independently of the chair, they would roll either toward (toe-in) or away (toe-out) from each other. Some wheel or caster adjustments can cause your wheels to be angled in one of these ways, making the chair harder to drive and possibly applying force on the frame and axles that can cause damage in the long term. When adding camber to your wheels, be sure to also look for toe-in or toe-out. Your technician needs to be sensitive to this issue.

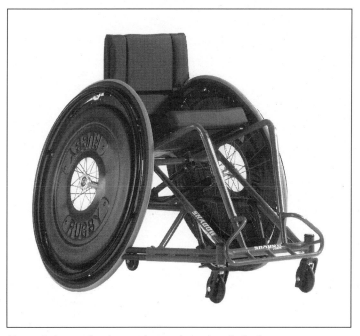

Figure 4. A specialized sport chair with cambered wheels

Handrims

The size of your hand will influence what size handrim should be used with a given size of wheel to ensure that you get the most efficiency in your push. The most common diameter of handrims is 20 or 21 inches. Handrims with a smaller radius from the axle require more force to propel the chair, just as a smaller gear on a bicycle makes it harder to pedal. Racing wheelchairs have very small rims because, once moving, the racer can keep his hands in contact with the rim to use the upward motion of his arms to continue to propel the chair. These rims make sense for providing continual motion during a race, but not for everyday use.

Many manual wheelers grasp both the tire and handrim simultaneously while they push. There are two advantages of using this "full-handed" technique. First, it helps you put more arm strength into the push since you don't need as much grasp force to hold both the tire and handrim as you would to grip only the rim. You are also less likely to overstrain muscles and tendons in the forearm. When gripping only the thin handrim, these muscles and tendons must work much harder to hold on. The "full-handed" wheeling technique is the reason that many chair riders have thick calluses on their palms, or wear fingerless gloves to protect their hands.

You will typically brake using the handrims. (Mounted brakes are for fixing the chair in place when you are stopped, not for slowing the chair while moving—that would put extreme wear on your tires.) Standard handrims are made of aluminum with an anodized, gray coating which is smooth enough not to burn your hands from friction as you brake, but not so slick that you can't slow yourself effectively with minimum grip force. Other options include plastic, foam, or powder coatings. These coatings increase the "grip-ability" of the handrim, but are more easily damaged. Plastic handrims can be very hot when braking and might seriously burn hands that lack sensation.

Handrims take a lot of abuse since they are the outermost surface of the chair. You will often navigate narrow spaces, so the rims will make a lot of contact with other surfaces, including door frames, metal shelves in stores, concrete surfaces, and other materials that will inevitably nick and scratch your handrims. You might as well get used to them getting scratched up if you are going to be active.

Standard handrims require a strong grip, but there are other designs that allow for less gripping ability. Low-level quadriplegic riders who use a manual chair can elect to use special handrims with added knobs which compensate for the wheeler's limited grip capacity. Some knobs project straight upward with no effect on the width of the chair, while others angle outward slightly to accommodate those with a limited ability to bend their hands at the wrist. A more aggressive option uses circular knobs about the size of a doorknob. The knobs are placed along the outside of the rim and rotate as you push against them while the wheel turns. This type of knob requires the least hand dexterity, but adds the most width to your chair.

Manual chair riders with only one arm can get a chair designed with a dual handrim on one wheel, allowing either or both wheels to be controlled with one hand.

Wheel locks

Wheel locks, also called hand brakes, are used to prevent a manual chair from accidentally rolling when you want it to remain stationary. Some chair riders have eschewed the use of brakes altogether, to the absolute horror of their therapists who subscribe to the belief that a wheelchair must be locked whenever you make a transfer to or from the chair. The instability of not having brakes can be dangerous.

The only people I have seen not use brakes are those that have very low level injuries and/or have some leg function. They can balance themselves well enough to transfer in and out of an unlocked chair. This doesn't work for me. The one (and only!) time I forgot to lock my brakes prior to a transfer I almost ended up on the ground, with the chair shooting off in the other direction!

There are other situations in which you'll be glad you have wheel locks. Just the act of reaching for an object on a table is enough to send sufficient force through your body to your wheels to cause the chair to shift, especially in a hypersensitive fixed-frame chair. If you are working at a desk, leaning forward on your arms will cause an unbraked chair to roll backward. Your wheels also give you the chance to discover that many floors are not level. It doesn't take much slope for you to roll downhill when you are in a well-maintained manual chair.

> I am mystified by how often I see people with no brakes, being so deeply in the habit of locking my chair whenever I am not in motion. This is not because I am so thoroughly brainwashed by my therapists from 25 years ago, but because I prefer the stability of a fixed seat that will not shift as I use my body.

Use of a hand brake also aids back support. Since you don't have to worry about the chair moving, you can rest your weight against the chair back with confidence.

People often don't have brakes because they are interested in removing as much weight as possible from their chair. Others are concerned about the danger of poking the end of their thumb on the brake as they wheel, a very painful experience indeed. When you wheel with the style of grabbing the tires and the handrim at the same time, your thumbs are more likely to hit the brake. Seat height also influences the likelihood of hitting your thumbs on the brake. When you sit lower, your arms will stroke farther down the wheels as you push and will be more likely to hit standard brakes.

A compromise solution is found in the "undermount" wheel locks, which are positioned beneath the wheelchair seat. These wheel locks are nowhere near your thumbs when you are pushing, but they are less convenient to operate, requiring you to lean forward and reach under the seat to engage them. Undermount wheel locks work best for people who have sufficient upper-body balance so that they only need to lock their wheels occasionally.

For those with limited hand and arm strength, extenders can be added to standard brake controls for additional leverage. Riders with extremely limited arm capacity might equip their chair with brakes an assistant can foot-operate from behind the chair.

Wheel locks installed too tightly to the chair can be very difficult to adjust or can possibly deform the frame, so make sure they are installed properly. If you use pneumatic tires, always set the brakes with the tires at their full capacity (maintain your tire pressure). The brakes get effectively looser as the tires get softer from losing air.

CHAPTER EIGHT

Power Chair Decisions

POWER WHEELCHAIRS HAVE COME A LONG WAY from the first models. The comfort and ease of driving a power chair have increased tremendously. No longer just a standard wheelchair with a motor added on, today's power chair is a complex, evolved, and integrated system that takes good advantage of modern manufacturing and computer technology.

Power chairs make a more active life on wheels possible for people who, in the past, would have been much more limited in their options and much more reliant on others for their mobility. People with progressive conditions also benefit a great deal from the ability to customize drive controls and other modular options as their needs change over time.

This chapter discusses the unique decisions to be made by those choosing a power chair. You need to get the right control system for you and the right kind of drive system. You need to think about speed—and about stopping. You need to decide which type and size of battery you want to use. Finally, you want to consider safety issues. Figure 5, "A rear-wheel drive, foldable power wheelchair," and Figure 6, "A front-wheel drive, elevating/reclining power wheelchair," show the various features found on power chairs and contrast some of the design differences.

Front-, rear-, or mid-wheel drive?

Power wheelchairs commonly have the drive wheels placed either at the front or the back of the chair. Mid-wheel drive is a relatively new alternative. Each type of wheel drive entails a different style of operating your chair, and takes a little while to adapt to the feel of it. If the type of drive is right for you, your skill and comfort using it will become increasingly refined, despite any early awkwardness you might experience.

With a front-wheel drive system, you have the sensation of pulling the chair behind you. This sense of pulling means that, in order to operate a front-wheel drive chair, you need greater sensitivity to the chair's movement and control. Front-wheel drive chairs are very agile—capable of making full rotations in a smaller area of space. But because front-wheel drive takes a little more skill to operate, ability and training issues must be taken into account. People with cognitive difficulties might not be able to safely use front-wheel drive.

One advantage of having the larger drive wheels in front is that you may be able to traverse a change in surface more easily—going over a curb, for example. The larger wheels make contact with the curb first, pulling the smaller casters along behind.

I live in a rural area where accessibility was initially the major issue. A chair with front-wheel drive would have better suited the terrain that I had to navigate.

If you need a tilt system, you will want to consider whether a front-wheel drive chair will be stable. The tilt system may cause the front wheels to come off the ground, making the chair difficult to operate.

When you operate a chair with rear-wheel drive, you feel as though you are being pushed forward. There is a greater sense of control over the chair, but rear-wheel drive doesn't afford as much agility.

Tipping is also a concern with rear-wheel drive. You may need to use anti-tippers with a rear-wheel drive chair, since it's possible for the casters in front to be lifted off the surface by the power and weight of the drive wheels in back when you accelerate the chair. The chair might also tend to tip if you are going up a steep incline. The position of the drive wheel axle also affects the possibility of tipping. The more forward the wheel, the more likely that the front casters will lift off the ground when you start to drive from a

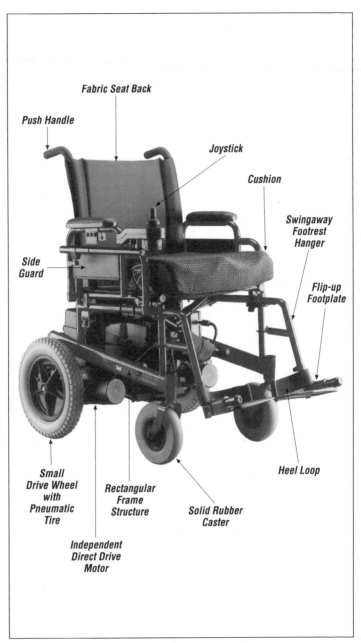

Fabric Seat Back

Push Handle

Joystick

Cushion

Swingaway
Footrest
Hanger

Side
Guard

Flip-up
Footplate

Small
Drive Wheel
with
Pneumatic
Tire

Rectangular
Frame
Structure

Independent
Direct Drive
Motor

Solid Rubber
Caster

Heel Loop

Figure 5. A rear-wheel drive, foldable power wheelchair

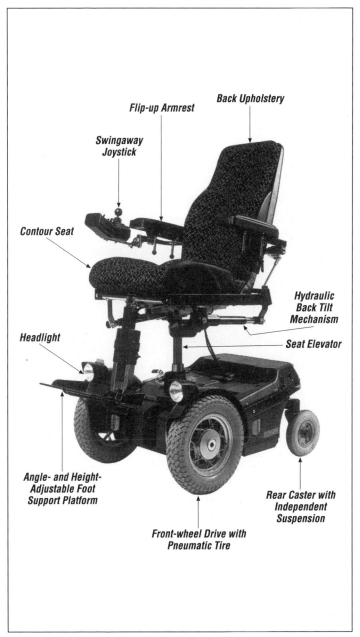

Swingaway Joystick

Flip-up Armrest

Back Upholstery

Contour Seat

Hydraulic Back Tilt Mechanism

Seat Elevator

Headlight

Angle- and Height-Adjustable Foot Support Platform

Front-wheel Drive with Pneumatic Tire

Rear Caster with Independent Suspension

Figure 6. A front-wheel drive, elevating/reclining power wheelchair

stopped position. Modern power chair controls allow you to specify how quickly acceleration occurs, so they compensate to some degree for the risk of tipping. Your goal is to find the best compromise between smooth acceleration and chair stability.

If the rear-wheel drive mechanism extends out of the rear of the chair and is low to the ground, you might have the opposite problem—not being able to tip back enough. This could limit your ability to climb over an obstacle or negotiate a ramp or curb cut.

A more recent alternative is the mid-wheel drive. The mid-wheel drive design uses six wheels: casters in the rear, the two drive wheels, and two more caster-size wheels in the front, which are not in continual contact with the ground but are there to help prevent forward tipping. These front casters are usually spring-loaded and adjustable.

The Jazzy wheelchair, from Pride Health Care, was the first mid-wheel drive chair, introduced in 1996. Invacare followed with several models.

The main advantage of mid-wheel drive is its tight turning radius. A mid-wheel drive chair can almost turn in place, making it helpful for people who must navigate small spaces at home or be able to turn around inside a van. For example, the Jazzy chair can turn in a radius of only 19.5 inches.

Mid-wheel drive helps to improve traction because more body weight is over the drive wheels, but there will always be some degree of forward tipping. Sudden stops or going forward down ramps are more likely to bring the front wheels in contact with the ground. Mid-wheel drives should be used only by people with good upper-body balance.

Mid-wheel drive chairs do best on firm surfaces. To use them on rough terrain, the front wheels need to be raised, and then more rocking occurs.

Comparison of Placement of Wheel Drive

Wheel drive placement	Advantages	Disadvantages
Front-wheel drive	Agile. Full rotations in smaller space. Easier to get over curbs.	More difficult to control. Not for those with cognitive disabilities. Less stable with tilt system.
Rear-wheel drive	Greater sense of control. Manufacturers have been. making longer, so design is well-refined.	Less agile. Front casters may come off the ground when accelerating.
Mid-wheel drive	Tight turning radius. Improved traction.	Requires good upper-body balance. Doesn't perform well on rough terrain.

Whichever placement of wheel drive you select, there will be a range of wheel sizes to choose from. The advantage of larger wheels is that they will enable you to drive more easily over changes in grade, possibly even small curbs. The disadvantage is that larger wheels add width to your chair. Use of independent suspension—which allows each wheel to shift upward with a change in surface—can make up for the loss of maneuverability in a chair with smaller wheels. (See Chapter 12, *Tires, Casters, and Suspension Systems*.)

Direct drive or belt drive?

The previous section dealt with issues to help you decide whether having the drive wheels in front, in back, or in the middle would make the most sense for the power chair you will drive. This section discusses the two different methods by which the wheels are made to turn, and how each affects the wheelchair operator.

One drive system for power chairs is direct drive. A direct drive system mounts the motor so that it turns gears, which directly mesh with the wheels. The other system is belt drive, which uses a belt to make the wheels turn. Direct drive has largely become the norm for power chairs. Few belt-driven chairs are being made anymore, but if you are thinking of buying a used chair or finding one through a charitable organization, you'll want to be aware of the differences between direct drive and belt drive.

Direct drive is popular because there are fewer parts, and therefore requires less maintenance. There are no belts to wear out. Direct drive takes better advantage of control technology. For instance, acceleration rates are easier to monitor and control with direct drive. Direct drive is also quieter.

The biggest disadvantage of direct drive systems is that they are less flexible. When there is a change in the terrain, the wheels can't adjust independently without losing contact with the gears. Some designs have overcome this problem with separate motors for each wheel, and independent suspension.

A belt drive system is naturally more flexible over changes in terrain because the belt is able to shift and continue to rotate the wheels. From a stopped position, there is a slight delay as tension builds in the belt before the wheels move, but this can mean a gentler start, with less of the jolt that could be a problem for a rider with limited upper-body balance. Some belt designs maintain a constant tension on the belts.

Belts, when wet, can lose their grip or slip off the drive wheel altogether. This power chair rider found the switch from belts made a beneficial difference:

> Belts break at the most inconvenient times. When they get wet, they slip. You have to time your stops precisely by letting off on the joystick at the right moment to avoid slippage. There's usually little tension on wet belts, so you'd better know exactly how much you can rely on before you get to the next curb cut, and you'd better get just the right amount of speed up before you try to get up a curb cut.

> Direct drive doesn't insist that I think about those things. It's always doing its job. My life isn't nearly as "adventurous" anymore.

One design, the HiRider from Falcon Rehabilitation, strikes a middle ground by using a chain instead of a belt. This frees the drive of the problems associated with flexible belts that might break.

Control systems

Power chair controls come in a number of designs and allow varying degrees of customization and programming.

Most power chair riders drive using a joystick control mounted on the armrest. The joystick should be positioned so that it can be comfortably reached by your dominant hand while you are sitting with good upright posture with your shoulders relaxed. Improper location of the joystick can mean that you have to compromise your posture in order to put your body in the right orientation to the control. If it is not accurately positioned, using the joystick can strain the hand and arm. If you need to sit close to a desk, you will need a joystick control that is able to swing away to the side. Not all joysticks are designed to do this.

For those unable to use a joystick, several other kinds of controls are available. There are breath controls (sometimes called sip-and-puff), which respond to an in or out breath, as if you were sucking on or blowing into a straw. Breath controls generally respond to more than one degree of pressure, so they can accept more than two commands. There are sanitary concerns, as the straws must be kept clean or replaced often.

Chin controls use a small rubber cup placed just below the chin. A chin control works essentially the same way as a joystick. Some people experience overuse strain in their neck or jaw muscles from the repetitive muscular exertion of using this type of control. There is some risk of temporomandibular joint disorder (TMJ), a chronic syndrome of muscle tightness and spasm in the facial muscles. The proper location and adjustment of the chin control are extremely important, as is sufficient training for the driver.

Another type of control employs head movements to the back and side, with nothing obstructing the face. Head controls rely heavily on computer programming. Their operation is not just a matter of pushing an object in the direction you want to move, as with a joystick. Head controls are also used for setting different modes, such as changing speed or reclining without making the chair move. A head control might even have an auxiliary setting that can open a door or answer the phone by remote control.

Parts of the control are in a headrest that responds to pressure applied with the back of the head. "Leaf switches," which can be sensitive to touch or head position, are located on either side of the headrest.

One man who has used both breath and chin controls prefers the head control because it gives him better vision range. He describes how his head control operates:

> If I push back against the headrest, then release, it sets the control to the slow speed mode. When I push back again, I go forward, controlling the speed with pressure up to a maximum speed set by the controller. (Mine is set to my girlfriend's walking speed.) If I apply pressure to my right, I steer right; the same with left. If I am in forward and hit the leaf switch beside my head, it puts me into reverse, and steering works the same way with movements of my head. Releasing pressure on the headrest brings the chair to a stop.

Obviously this is a control that requires some training to use. It might not be appropriate for people with cognitive disabilities who would have trouble remembering and quickly applying the variety of options available.

Karl Ylonen of Care Corporation offers his view of control systems:

> I always try to make a system as clean as I can. I don't like to use chin controls or sip-and-puff. They obstruct your vision, block your face from others. They are probably the last option for most people. That said, I see people who use sip-and-puff and love it. It works really well for them.

The integrated circuit has allowed power chair controls to become quite sophisticated. Modern controls allow customization of such functions as:

- Maximum speed.

- Minimum speed.

- Acceleration rate.

- Braking rate.

- Throw distance of control handle.

- Sensitivity of control handle.

For people who do not have steady hands, the sensitivity control allows the joystick to ignore sudden movements in the case of spasms, shaky hands, or rough terrain. The chair will maintain steady forward movement.

Setting the controls initially and making changes to them needs to be done by a qualified technician. (Some chairs allow multiple settings the user can choose from. See the section "How fast?" later in this chapter.) The safety of the user is a primary concern, although some experienced users prefer the convenience of being able to adjust control settings themselves.

My experience in purchasing a power chair was that the user is unable to make adjustments to any of the computerized controls themselves because a separate programming module is required that only a technician has.

Some controls are supplied with a selection of pre-set programs for learners at various stages and abilities, sip-and-puff users, and so on. The programming device can sometimes be used to perform diagnostics to ensure that the controls are working properly, to make fine adjustments to individual functions, or report battery levels. Invacare recently introduced a chair in its Action line that can be checked over the telephone through a computer modem by a technician in their factory.

The settings of your control are crucial, and you will need to work with a competent technician who understands your activities and needs. If you set too slow a deceleration rate, for example, but don't have sufficient dexterity or skill level, you might find yourself running into your furniture a lot because the chair keeps rolling once you have let go of the joystick. In this sense, the added capabilities of the technology also bring along certain potential risks. These risks will be offset by working with skilled folks who know how to match physical abilities to chair control choices, and by being well trained yourself in using the chair.

Electronics are in many ways the weak link in power chairs. Electronics generate heat, so the control unit can be burned out from overuse. You will need to gain a sense of the limits of your control unit. It can handle only so many hours of continuous use. Many power riders make a habit of switching off the power at the control unit to let it cool. New designs are beginning to incorporate a heat sink into the design that will prevent internal components from overheating.

How fast?

Safety should be the most important consideration when determining maximum speed. Remember that a power chair is not a motorcycle. It is not built for the road. You don't register it at your local Department of Motor Vehicles and get a license plate (although there are probably a few power chair riders who wish they could use the open road, given how difficult it can be to use public transportation).

What will happen if you are going fast and a dog or a child suddenly steps out in front of you? A sudden stop might throw you out of your chair if you do not have sufficient upper-body balance or are riding without the use of restraints. You might also lose your grasp of the controller in such a situation. Both maximum speed and stopping distance (deceleration) can be programmed in modern controllers, and you would be well advised to err on the side of your own safety—as well as that of anyone who might accidentally get in your way.

A safe and comfortable maximum speed depends on where you are, particularly whether you're inside or outside.

For use indoors, a maximum speed of five miles per hour is a recommended standard. When you are inside, moving in smaller spaces, a slow speed can feel fast. Traveling the short distance from your desk at work to the bathroom, or from your living room to your kitchen, seems to go quickly even though you may actually be moving slowly.

A speed that is comfortable inside feels slow once you are out on the sidewalk. Outside, you usually travel farther, and you are more conscious of how long it takes to reach your destination. Traveling from your home to the corner grocery store four blocks away can seem like an eternity using the same speed you were using inside your home.

Yet outside you might be with another person who walks. Walking speed always seems slow to a wheelchair rider, yet you don't want to make your companions run to keep up with you. Average walking speed is three miles per hour, whereas a moderate running pace is eight miles per hour, numbers you can take into account when choosing your chair. Some chairs are capable of traveling as fast as eight miles per hour.

User definition of speed is now typical of power chairs and scooters. A common feature of modern power controls is a switch that lets you alternate between two programs so you can have a maximum indoor speed and a higher maximum outdoor speed. Another approach is a knob that allows you to adjust maximum speed. Some manufacturers are concerned about liability issues in allowing user changes. They have intentionally designed their controls to require more steps to change maximum speed. This can mean an additional level of safety for users, but many find the extra safeguards inconvenient and unnecessary.

How you stop your power chair depends on whether you have belt or direct drive. The advent of direct drive made automatic brakes possible, since there is enough "grip" between the gears and the wheels to hold the chair firmly in place. A belt drive system will always slip some on a slope, and drivers find that to hold themselves in place they must actually apply backward drive or else manually apply wheel brakes.

One rider who went from using belt drive to direct drive explains the difference:

> I didn't think I'd like auto-braking at all. With my E & J chairs, the only way to stop was to go into reverse. That provided a lot more control over whether you came to a slow, easy stop or an abrupt one. But the computerized controller on my new Quickie P300 was able to be adjusted so that I didn't have to worry about abrupt stops; auto-braking has won me over quite thoroughly. It's nice to be able to stop on a slope and not have to manually set the brakes or keep my hand on the joystick.

Anyone changing to a power chair after being used to a manual chair will find automatic braking a little odd. You become accustomed to coasting in a manual chair. With automatic braking, if you are not pushing on that stick, you aren't going anywhere. But if you find yourself on sloped surfaces often, it's a godsend.

Types of batteries

There are two primary types of batteries used for power chairs: gel cell and lead acid—also called wet cell. There are also different battery sizes, which are discussed in the next section, "Battery power." When you buy a chair, you choose the type and capacity of the batteries. For some chairs, the battery is a separate item, not included in the price of the standard package.

Batteries are commonly found items that need not be purchased from a wheelchair supplier, and might, in fact, be found at better prices from other battery supply sources. You do not want to buy automobile batteries, however. The voltage needed to start a six-cylinder engine is much different from what your wheelchair needs. Also, car batteries are designed for a quick release of energy, whereas wheelchair batteries provide "continuous deep discharging" or "deep-cycle" power.

Gel cell batteries are currently more the norm. You will pay a bit more for gel batteries, but they require less maintenance since you don't have to put water in them or worry about acid spills. Gel batteries don't last as long as wet cells and are slightly less powerful. But gel battery technology has improved, and the gap between their capacity and that of wet cell batteries is closing.

Wet cell batteries can be charged more times than the gel type, and so have a longer life span. Longer life makes wet cell batteries preferable for very active users who would otherwise need to replace expensive batteries more often.

Wet cell batteries require more maintenance, though. It is necessary to maintain their water level. They are susceptible to leaking or spilling acid. Most airlines will not allow wet cell batteries on an airplane because they contain hazardous material. You can now find sealed lead acid batteries that solve some of these problems—they are maintenance-free and are much less likely to leak.

Battery power

You will need to choose not only the type of battery best suited to your needs, but also the most appropriate battery size.

Battery power is rated in amp-hours. The higher the number of amp-hours, the more power and the longer it will last. Amp-hour ratings are generally about ten percent higher for wet cells than for gel batteries.

There are three sizes of batteries used for adult chairs. Group 22 batteries are the standard size, but Group 24 batteries are used as standard equipment for heavier, high performance chairs. Group 24 batteries are often offered as an option by the manufacturer. Group 27 batteries—at 105 amp-hours for the wet cells—are the powerhouse units. You might need this largest size if you really plan to go the distance.

How far your power chair or scooter can travel depends not only on battery type and size, but other factors as well. The heavier your chair, the more battery power it will use. Larger drive wheels take less power than small ones. If you climb a lot of slopes, even gentle ones, your chair will have to work much harder. In hilly San Francisco, one needs more battery power than in a level place like Des Moines, Iowa.

You will also place a greater demand on your need for power if you tend to have a racier driving style. And obviously, someone working at a desk job will find their batteries lasting much longer than a supervisor who travels the factory floor all day. The farther you go in a day, the more you climb hills, and the more equipment you have on your chair (such as a tilt and recline system), the more power you will need.

It is extremely important that you not risk losing battery power at critical times, such as when traveling away from home or on a cold winter night. Battery power can be a life or death matter, so you must ensure you have sufficient power for your needs and that you keep your batteries charged and well maintained.

In the event that you do have a battery or mechanical failure, you want the ability to disengage the drive system so someone can push the chair manually. You might even prefer this option to allow yourself the choice of being pushed over certain types of terrain. It should not require an advanced engineering degree to switch to manual mode. One simple design uses a knob that you simply pull and rotate slightly to release the wheels from the drive mechanism.

Battery chargers

It's important to take the time to identify the right batteries for your needs, because you will also be buying a battery charger. Most chargers are made for specific types and ratings of batteries. If you switch to another battery group size, or from wet cell to gel batteries, you will probably have to spend money for a different charger as well.

You will want an automatic charger, capable of shutting itself off when the battery has reached its full capacity. Manual chargers continue to charge, and can damage your batteries if you don't unplug them on time. Even automatic chargers continue to release small amounts of energy, and should not be left on for more than 24 hours.

You might want to have the flexibility to change battery types. For example, you might want the extra power of wet cell batteries for daily activities, but need to use gel cell batteries for traveling. Some battery charger manufacturers provide products that might be of interest to wheelchair owners who use more than one kind of battery.

The Soneil SuperCharger is designed to be used for both gel and wet cell batteries. This "switch-mode" charger comes with connectors for most major wheelchair brands, and can be used with either 110 current or the 220-volt current used in Europe. The SuperCharger takes a bit more time to charge than a specialized charger for your type of battery, but you might not mind trading the extra time in order to gain more flexibility than the standard charger offers. Make sure the charger settings for different battery types are not too easy to change, lest they become switched to the wrong type by accident. Charging your batteries at the wrong setting can cause severe damage to your chair or even risk starting a fire.

Another interesting product is the Battery Booster from D & D Advanced Technologies. It charges the standard 24-volt batteries power chairs use, but is also capable of providing 12-volt power for accessories you might want to have with your chair. You can power a small television, a CB radio or cellular phone, a CD player, and so on. If you drive, this charger can also extend the amount of power available in a given day by allowing you to charge your batteries from the cigarette lighter receptacle in your van.

Safety

Power wheelchairs have some potentially dangerous moving parts and electrical connections that need to be properly shielded. A curious child might want to explore the inner workings of your chair, or a weak leg or arm can unintentionally slip and get caught in a gear or switch. These areas should be sufficiently covered, but in a way that does not make it unduly difficult to service your chair. Be sure that your clothes cannot possibly get caught in any moving parts.

You must be confident that you could not possibly receive an electric shock and that you won't lose control of your chair. The ANSI/RESNA standards encourage that:

- The chair frame should not be electrically grounded so it cannot transmit electric current to your body.

- It should be impossible to touch any uninsulated parts.

- Wiring should not be able to be connected incorrectly.

- The controller should be resistant to damage should there be an improper wiring connection.

- The chair should not be driveable while the battery is charging.

- Surfaces of the wheelchair should never become heated from the electrical system.

- Failure of the electrical system should not result in uncontrolled movement of the chair.

Operating your power chair in severe weather can have an effect on the electronics of your chair. Major changes in temperature—whether going from air conditioning into the sun or from a heated building into winter weather—can put a lot of stress on your control systems. ANSI/RESNA prescribes tests for the effects of both temperature change and rain on a power chair, using a pass/fail basis, the results of which should appear on the product literature. Testers literally put the chair into a shower, expose it to extreme cold or heat before a driving test, and check performance once the chair has returned to room temperature.

CHAPTER NINE

Cushions

ALTHOUGH YOUR WHEELCHAIR AND CUSHION are separate purchases, which chair you choose is significantly affected by the type of cushion you will use. Chair and cushion are a team, each influencing the other. The proper combination of chair and cushion will enable you to sit in a neutral and stable position and to operate the chair safely.

Cushions come in various depths and sizes, which need to be accommodated by the size of your wheelchair frame. The actual length of footrests, the height of the chair back, the position of armrests, and other features are influenced by how high or low you will be sitting on a cushion. Clearly, you need to decide which cushion is best for you before you can make a final decision about which chair is best, and certainly before you specify the exact dimensions of your chair.

Wheelchair cushion development is quite lively, as designers and engineers continue the quest for the ideal cushion. A number of manufacturers, such as Jay and Roho, exist solely for the design and production of seating and support systems for wheelchairs. Most of the major wheelchair makers, including Everest & Jennings, Invacare/Pindot, and Otto Bock Reha, also offer an assortment of cushions.

Cushion design is by no means a simple topic, and there are many choices to make as you decide on the right one for you. This chapter discusses the four basic types of cushions—foam, gel, air flotation, and urethane honeycomb—as well as designs and systems for more specialized needs.

Cushion function

What kind of cushion you choose will depend on a variety of factors, including how much time you spend in your chair, how much you move around in your chair, and how stable your posture is.

One important task of the wheelchair cushion is the prevention of pressure sores. Since, when we sit, only one third of the body's surface is supporting all of its weight, blood flow is restricted. In the presence of muscle atrophy—which is experienced in particular by many people with spinal cord injuries—circulation is limited further by the loss of muscle, which once served as a sort of natural cushion. An additional risk of sitting is shear force, as we tend to slide forward in the cushion, causing stress across the surface of the skin. Resulting pressure sores (decubitus ulcers) can be very serious, leading to hospitalization, surgery, and—although rare—even death. The right cushion is a primary tool for maintaining the health of your skin.

The other crucial task for a cushion is postural stability. Even if you are able to walk or are an amputee with sufficient built-in cushioning, the right cushion helps to support your spine. If you already have some asymmetry in your body, you need to be supported in a way that will not increase any spinal deformity. For manual chair users, greater stability in your chair also means you can push the wheels with more confidence and strength.

It can't be repeated often enough—posture is key. Bob Hall of New Hall's Wheels puts it well:

> *The wrong seating system leads to poor posture, which leads to physical problems, which lead to becoming more sedentary, which leads to a negative emotional and personal experience. It's a dangerous chain of events.*

Foam cushions

Foam technology has come a long way. No longer just the soft, airy stuff of the past, foam now comes in a range of densities and with varying degrees of "memory," holding its shape as you sit, contributing to your stability. The new foams can adapt to any shape and still provide even support, spreading pressure across the sitting surface. Different foams are often used in combination, layered for their various properties of softness, even support, and memory.

Foam is relatively inexpensive, and it is easy to cut. A therapist can experiment with shapes free of financial risk. If you have an area of skin that is broken down or on the verge, pressure can easily be reduced by cutting out a portion of the cushion. (You should not do this on your own, though, because only a doctor or therapist can identify the changes in your cushion that will help relieve pressure while still maintaining appropriate support.)

On the downside, foam wears out faster than other materials and loses its shape, but because of its lower price, this might not concern you. If you choose a foam cushion, be sure to replace it when its time is up. Old foam that is compressed can allow pressure points to form that can lead to a sore.

If you choose a gel or air flotation cushion for daily use, it is a good idea to have a backup foam cushion, since gel and air flotation cushions can leak.

Gel cushions

Gel cushion designs attempt, in effect, to replace the consistency and support of atrophied muscle tissue. Highly engineered gel fluids are placed in pouches and usually attached to a foam base, so that the cushion conforms to the pressures placed on it. As a result, gel cushions provide excellent pressure distribution and are very comfortable. Many gel products also offer supplemental inserts to stabilize your legs. Your knees might tend to fall together (adduction) or apart (abduction), so such an accessory can help keep your legs straight, which also aids your overall posture.

Unfortunately, gel cushions are much heavier than other types, which can cancel out some of the benefits of your lightweight wheelchair. Gel suppliers such as Jay and Flofit offer lighter, active-use designs, but these might not be appropriate for you if you are unable to do your own pressure-relief lifts.

If you bounce up and down curbs, or commonly experience similar impact in your chair, a gel cushion might not be ideal. When you sit in a gel cushion, there is no further "cushiness" to absorb impact, a concept known as impact loading. Other cushion types are better able to absorb impact.

Another drawback to gel cushions is the possibility of them "bottoming out" as the gel is pushed aside by your weight. You can help prevent this distribution problem by kneading your gel cushion once a day, keeping the fluids loose and spread evenly. Look for a design that divides the gel portion into several sections so that all of the gel cannot push to the sides.

There is also the chance of the gel leaking. While cushions arrive with patching kits, patches are ineffective when the breach is at a seam, which is often the case. A leak might be very minor, or it could be an extremely messy affair.

Air or dry flotation cushions

Air flotation cushions support the body entirely on air. A typical example is the Roho cushion, designed with a group of small, interconnected rubber balloons arranged in rows. Pressure is balanced by air shifting out to surrounding balloons, spreading pressure evenly against your skin. The whole system is closed, so air flotation cushions can't bottom out the way gel cushions can.

If you have a pressure sore, you can tie off individual balloons to reduce contact under that area, allowing you to spend more time sitting as the sore heals. The Roho Quadtro allows the user to inflate four quadrants separately for optimal positioning. Air cushions are relatively lightweight and are waterproof, allowing for double duty in the bathtub or on a boat.

Crown Therapeutics, maker of the Roho cushions, also offers air flotation products for the wheelchair back, supplemental lumbar or sacral support, full bed cushions, and even a product for a standard toilet seat. All are inflatable to adjust to your needs.

A longtime presence in disability magazines has been an ad for the "Bye-Bye Decubiti" cushion. It is inflatable, comes in many different sizes and shapes, is made of heavy-duty rubber, and—although different from the Roho balloon design—is uniquely formed to minimize pressure at the bony protrusions on which we sit.

Air cushions can be less stable for those who move around a lot in their chair, but recent designs offer either low profile or quadrant options that minimize this problem. The balloons used in air cushions can be punctured, of course, and leaks do occur, although a fairly heavy-duty rubber is used. But patching them is easier than with the gel design. The hard part is submerging the cushion under water to find the leak (look for escaping air bubbles).

The biggest drawback to air cushions is that they require more maintenance. It is necessary to check the pressure frequently, especially if you have pressure sores.

Urethane honeycomb cushions

Thermoplastic urethane honeycomb cushions are the most recent development in the world of cushions. Because there are many individual cells—like a beehive—these cushions are able to distribute weight evenly, but there is no risk of leaking gel or of an air bladder being punctured. The many open spaces in the beehive structure of the cushion allow air to travel more effectively. This design helps to protect against skin breakdown because your skin is kept cooler and moisture is prevented from collecting.

Urethane honeycomb cushions are very light and absorb shock, and a low-profile cushion can provide significant support. These cushions can even be thrown into your washing machine and dryer, making them attractive for people with incontinence problems, where the cushion will be soiled from time to time despite best efforts at bowel and bladder management.

Supracor of San Jose, California, makes several honeycomb cushions based on their patent. One type uses multiple layers of varying stiffness to allow your sit bones to sink into the cushion while deeper layers provide overall support and weight distribution. Another type is contoured to provide adduction and abduction, plus a rear dish for pelvic positioning. There is not much of a track record for urethane honeycomb cushions because of their recent development, but there appear to be good prospects for this type of cushion to evolve and become more widely used.

Comparison of Main Types of Cushions

Cushion type	Advantages	Disadvantages
Foam	Inexpensive. Very lightweight. Comes in range of densities. Holds shape (memory). Provides even support. Can be cut to relieve sores. Nothing to leak	Wears out faster. Loses its shape. Old, compressed foam could lead to a sore.
Gel	Excellent pressure distribution. Very comfortable. May have supplemental inserts to stabilize legs.	Heavy. Chance of leakage. Less able to absorb impact. Some designs allow gel to push out to sides.
Air flotation	Lightweight. Even pressure distribution. Will not bottom out if properly inflated. Can be modified to relieve pressure sores. Some models inflate to user's specific needs. Waterproof.	Less stable. Chance of puncture/leakage. High maintenance: need to check pressure frequently.

Comparison of Main Types of Cushions (continued)

Urethane honeycomb	Very lightweight Low profile in appearance. Distributes weight evenly. Good support. Absorbs shock. Keeps skin cooler. No risk of leakage. Machine washable/dryable.	Relatively new, so not much of a track record yet.

Alternating pressure

The latest territory being explored in cushion design is the use of an air pump to create alternating pressure, of particular interest to those with more severe disabilities who are unable to perform their own weight shifts to relieve pressure.

Sitting for extensive periods of time without pressure relief causes the muscle and fatty tissues to separate, putting the delicate skin layer in closer contact with the bone. This creates even more pressure on the skin. Lack of air circulation increases the temperature between you and the cushion. Moisture collects and is trapped against the skin. All of this further increases the risk of a sore.

One alternating pressure solution is the ErgoDynamic Seating System from ErgoAir in New Hampshire. This system pumps air into and out of alternating portions of the cushion. The product is contoured for pelvic stability, with a pre-ischial cross-bar design that prevents forward slipping—and therefore shear—on the cushion. Special vent holes serve to allow the flow of air and moisture. In a five-minute cycle, compartments are inflated and deflated to shift support alternately between the ischial (sit) bones and the hips. Both areas get regular periods of complete pressure relief. The manufacturer likens it to a massage while you sit, with the resulting promotion of blood flow. In some cases, the makers suggest, a pressure sore can even heal while you sit. This cushion system can be plugged into some power chair batteries or charged in a cigarette lighter in your car.

Alternating pressure products are of course heavier—given their use of batteries and air pumps—and, like air flotation cushions, prone to puncture. However, the technology for these innovative systems is likely to evolve further in the future, as new materials and batteries are developed.

Positioning systems

Advanced needs such as significant spinal curvatures or asymmetries in your body require more complex kinds of trunk support. For example, the Pindot system, recently acquired by Invacare and available from suppliers around the country, is a support system that customizes seat and back cushions to your exact shape. First, a special chair takes an imprint of your body's shape. A therapist views a computer image of the shape and can customize the contours of your cushion. From your imprint and the therapist's specifications, a foam cushion that gives you optimal support is manufactured specifically for you. The Pindot system is of most value to people who will not move around much in their chair. Since the cushion is formed to your shape, you will only be comfortable in it when you sit in the right relationship to the customized contours.

Your needs might require the services of a rehab engineer who custom designs your seating system. A rehab engineer might adapt existing products or build something from scratch just for you. Your therapist or dealer should be aware of such people in your area. Often they are working in a major hospital or university. The Veteran's Administration is also involved in research and engineering that addresses the need for customized positioning systems.

More information about positioning systems can be found in the section "Lateral supports" in Chapter 13, *Tilt/Recline Systems and Positioning Systems*.

CHAPTER TEN

Seats and Backs

ALTHOUGH WE USUALLY THINK OF A SEAT as a single unit—such as a couch or recliner—seats, backs, cushions, and armrests are distinct when you are choosing your wheelchair. Seats, backs, and cushions have a number of interrelationships, so to some degree, you will need to think about them all at the same time. For instance, how high you will sit on the chair will be determined by the seat-to-floor height of the seat pan plus the thickness of the cushion.

The previous chapter was devoted to cushions. Armrests are optional and are discussed in Chapter 14, *Armrests, Clothing Guards, and Accessories*.

This chapter will help you understand the proper dimensions for the seat and back of your chair. We discuss various considerations for choosing the width, depth, and angle of the seat, as well as how high your seat will be from the ground. We also explain options for back support, back height, and back angle. Finally, this chapter discusses whether to include push handles on the back of the chair.

Seat/chair width

Your chair should be as narrow as possible for your body size without creating contact points that can cause pressure sores.

A seat that is too wide limits mobility. A quarter of an inch in the width of the chair can make the difference between being able to get down an aisle in a store or past a couch at the home of a friend. You don't want to squeeze yourself into the seat—if you wear a heavy coat in the winter, or typically work in a business suit with a jacket, the width of the seat should take this into account—but you also don't need the wasted space or mobility limitations of a chair that is too wide. A wider chair is also heavier, given the extra metal in the frame.

A seat that is too wide will promote poor posture. If you have extra space, you are more likely to slump to one side or the other. You might think that, because you would have more room to shift your position, extra seat width would be helpful in the prevention of pressure sores, but this is not a good strategy for skin management. You don't want to protect your skin by risking damage to your spine with twisted sitting postures. Rather, your skin management program should consist of proper cushioning and diet, as well as push-ups while you are in the chair. Put a high priority on good postural habits.

A wider chair also means that the wheels will be wider apart, making it necessary for a manual chair wheeler to reach farther, extending arms out to the side. Wheeling with arms extended is a less efficient way to wheel and will be more fatiguing. If the chair has armrests, they might further interfere with the process of wheeling if the chair is too wide for you, or rub against your arms as you wheel.

A wider chair does provide better lateral stability, which will help prevent a manual chair from tipping over sideways, but frankly, unless you are reckless or wheel on rough terrain, tipping sideways isn't likely. Stability can be similarly achieved by proper adjustment of the axles and plates that are typical on most chairs today. The wheels can be moved out and camber added for stability without having to incur the disadvantages and risks of a wider frame.

If weight management is difficult for you, you will want to take the possibility of weight gain into consideration when determining the seat width. You don't want to find yourself ultimately squeezed into a chair purchased when you were lighter. Your risk of pressure sores—particularly at your hip bones—will increase considerably. If you become heavier and truly need a new chair, you might have to fight with your funding source for approval, or be forced to dip into your own savings or credit limit to buy new wheels. But do you want to purchase a wider chair on the assumption that you will gain weight? Is that risking a self-fulfilling prophesy, inviting weight gain? The best solution is to reach a stable weight, whatever is normal for you, and then specify a chair that will remain appropriate to your needs while you practice the best weight control habits you can.

Seat depth

It is critical to get the depth of the seat pan right when you specify the dimensions of your chair. The seat pan should be deep enough so that the seat is in contact with as much of the bottom of your thighs as possible.

When the seat pan is too shallow, your upper legs extend beyond the front edge and more pressure is placed on your ischial "sitting" bones. This additional pressure increases the risk of skin breakdown. You are also giving up greater stability. The chair can't "carry" you if it can't make full contact with your body. Without full seat support, your body might be prevented from being in its neutral position, risking spinal curvature or muscle and tendon strain. A too-shallow seat pan also means that your feet will not rest properly in the footrests.

On the other hand, when the seat pan is too deep, you will be unable to sit properly against the chair back. You will be kept from sliding back fully in the seat, stopped behind the knees. When the seat is too deep, the only way to make contact with the back of the chair is to rotate the pelvis backward and round the spine. In other words, you will have to slump. Slumping is potentially dangerous for the spine as it can cause degeneration. This posture also makes it difficult for you to wheel efficiently in a manual chair.

A seat pan that is too deep can interfere with the position of your legs if you use calf supports with your footrests. Calf supports keep the legs in a more forward position. The seat pan might need to be shallower to compensate.

A deeper seat means a heavier chair due to the added metal in the frame. When more of the chair is ahead of the axle, you will feel as though you are pushing even more weight. If you require extra depth in the seat pan, you will need to adjust the forward position of the main wheel axles so the chair is not too front-heavy, particularly if you rely on doing wheelies in your wheeling style.

> I am very tall, and recently purchased a chair that is two inches deeper than my past wheels so I could have more contact with my legs along the seat. It has worked very well, and it was not a problem to adjust the chair for wheelies and for ease of wheeling, although it did feel slightly heavier at first. Now I can't tell the difference, partly because I have nothing to compare to anymore, and I probably gained a little strength to compensate for the additional weight just by using the chair.

A crucial element that must be taken into consideration before you can determine the appropriate depth of the seat pan is the type of seat back you will use. A fabric-upholstered back requires you to sit a little farther back in the chair, and tends to loosen with time unless it is equipped with adjustable tension straps. A rigid back will not change much over time, but some are quite thick and cause you to sit more forward on the seat.

Seat height

The minimum height you can sit off the ground will be determined by physical factors. The main considerations are the length of your legs and the clearance needed for footrests. Whether you'll choose to sit higher than the minimum—and how much higher—will depend on environment, such as the height of standard tables or other surfaces, and on personal preferences.

The seat-to-floor height of a manual chair will be part of the frame dimensions ordered from the factory. It can also be controlled by where the axle plates are installed relative to the supports that carry the seat sling—the lower the axle plates, the higher the seat. On a modular power chair, the seat structure is installed on top of a drive unit and so does not depend as much on the wheel position. Instead, seat height is determined by the structure that holds the seat, which might be adjustable or be available from the manufacturer in a choice of heights.

The minimum seat height for your wheelchair is determined by how much space your footrests need to clear the floor. How high you sit and how long your legs are determine where your feet will end up. In calculating minimum footrest clearance, you need to account for bumps in sidewalks, table leg supports, or any other kinds of changes in the surface you might encounter to determine how high your footrests should be from the ground. ANSI/RESNA recommends two inches of clearance from the ground for footrests, but depending on where you will be riding, you might need more.

Whether you want your seat to be higher than the minimum height depends on a number of factors. The higher you sit, the better you can reach your cabinets in the kitchen, shelves in stores, or a book-shelf at work. Your visibility will also be a little better. Be sure, though, that your knees will be able to fit under tables and desks. On the other hand, it might be important for you to be closer to the floor, perhaps for your work. You might need to be at the same level as the surfaces you transfer to, such as your car seat or your bed. If you are a manual chair rider, you want to consider how far you will have to reach to push your wheels. Remember to add the thickness of your cushion to determine how high you will actually sit in your chair.

If you sit too low, you might strain your neck in conversation with people who are standing next to you. Some people feel that, when they sit low, they are less charismatic or appear inferior to those around them. They feel "looked down upon." However, seat height preference is an individual matter. Some folks are just happier at a higher—or lower—level. Make sure you take time to consider all the practical, psychological, and personal aspects that will be affected by the height of your chair.

Seat angle

Your chair seat does not necessarily need to be parallel to the ground. Seats can slope down toward the back. The angle of the seat compared to the ground is sometimes called "seat dump" or "squeeze." (See Figure 4, "A specialized sport chair with cambered wheels," in Chapter 7, *Manual Chair Decisions*, for an example of extreme seat dump.)

Having some degree of seat dump means that more of your weight presses against the chair back, making you feel more stable in your seat. People with higher level spinal disabilities gain security and safety with the use of seat dump. Manual riders are able to exert more push with less effort through their arms and shoulders.

Many chairs are designed so you can adjust seat dump. The advent of rigid-frame designs made it easier to adjust the angle of the seat, since the seat support rails are no longer part of the chair's folding mechanism. On a folding chair, these rails are fixed, so the seat angle is determined by the position of the axles relative to the entire frame. Raising the rear axles to a higher position has the effect of lowering the rear of the chair and so increases the seat dump. It might also be possible to raise the caster height, achieving the same effect.

There are trade-offs for the advantages of seat dump:

- When your knees are raised relative to your thighs, the pelvis rotates backward with your legs, and the spine is flexed into a rounded shape, flattening out the lumbar curve, which plays an important role in the health of your spine. Too much dump, therefore, can increase the risk of scoliosis or disk problems, so should not be used to an extreme. If you experience back pain after using more seat angle, you should adjust it toward a more level angle.

- Your therapist must make sure you have sufficient flexibility to bend at the hips for added seat dump. Closing the hip angle too much can limit circulation to the legs, already at risk of circulation difficulties from not being used.

- Seat dump can increase shear forces if you are not sitting back fully in the chair with a proper cushion. Also, your therapist and dealer should make sure there is not too much pressure on the sacral bone at the base of your spine, a common site of pressure sores. Some backs and cushions are designed to reduce sacral pressure.

- Finally, a more pronounced seat dump might make it more difficult for you to transfer in and out of your chair.

Back support

Until recently, cloth or vinyl sling backs, which necessarily had to fold with the chair, were the only choice. Flat backs provided no lumbar support, lateral trunk stability, or accommodation of people with more advanced orthopedic/neurologic needs.

Aware of the need for better postural support, chair and cushion designers directed their efforts to making other options available. A back that must fold with the chair is much less an issue now. Rigid-frame chairs use a back that pivots down against the seat, rather than closing sideways. Power chairs designed in modules are not made to fold, so the back can now be designed with more shape, support, and upholstered comfort.

One current back design that can still close with a folding chair enhances the traditional cloth back by adding a series of horizontal looped straps down the outside of the chair back. (See Figure 7, "A chair back with tension-adjustable straps.") The straps are tension-adjustable so that each strap can be individually tightened or loosened according to the need for support at a particular point in your back. For instance, the strap behind the point where the chair back needs to support your lumbar curve is usually pulled tighter than the strap behind the top of the back. This combination of adjustments optimizes even contact with the seat back all the way up your back while helping you maintain the best possible posture. It is not always possible to accomplish ideal posture with a strapped-back design, but this kind of enhancement offers much better support than a flat back alone.

A more recent development in the attempt to provide lumbar support for sling-back wheelchairs is the PaxBac from Invacare/Pin-Dot. The PaxBac is positioned at your lumbar curve and typically provides more support than a tension back. It is made of molded foam and is designed so that support is applied on either side of the spine. (This allows the shape of the PaxBac to be narrow in the middle so that it can fold with the wheelchair.) You control the amount of back support with a strap system that attaches to the upright canes of the chair. The key to the design is the ease of operating the strap—with a simply released "cam buckle"—while you are sitting in the chair. The PaxBac will, however, add about two pounds to the weight of your chair.

Another approach to back support is a rigid back with deep upholstery. These products typically allow you to adjust lumbar support. To install this kind of chair back, the standard cloth back is removed entirely, support clips are added to the vertical canes of the chair, and the new back is hung on these clips. For a folding chair, this back must be lifted off before the chair can be folded. The decision to choose a back of this design will probably depend

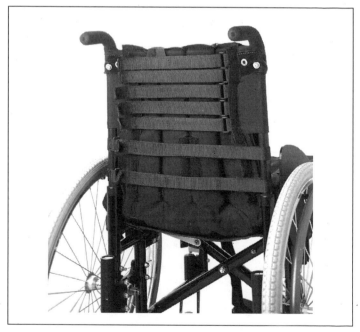

Figure 7. A chair back with tension-adjustable straps

on cost and/or the potential inconvenience of having to remove the back. The design comes in a variety of sizes and heights.

If you will be pushing a manual chair, you'll want to weigh the benefits of greater back support against the additional weight of a more supportive back. Keep in mind that with extra back support you will be able to maintain more firm contact with the back of the chair as you push, enabling you to exert more force on the wheels.

If your strength and balance are more limited, your need for other back support features increases. For instance, if you have limited side-to-side stability, you can choose a back cushion that wraps around you, curving to your sides to help support you laterally. (See Figure 8, "A deep contour back.") If your balance is precarious or you tend to slip easily from neutral posture, you might require additional lateral support accessories or a hip and/or chest seat belt.

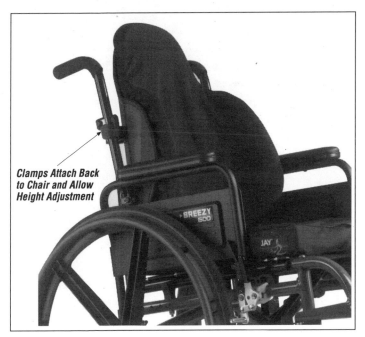

Clamps Attach Back to Chair and Allow Height Adjustment

Figure 8. A deep contour back

Chapter 13, *Tilt/Recline Systems and Positioning Systems*, has more information about additional support for those who need more help with stability.

For people whose bodies are not symmetrical, the chair back might need to be customized by a rehabilitation engineer who works closely with your therapist and wheelchair supplier. This more advanced approach can involve making molds of your body to make a highly specialized support system specifically for your needs.

Back height

You need sufficient support for your lower and upper back. Your balance may be limited by being unable to use your legs. If you are paralyzed as high as your abdomen and trunk, you are not able to use those muscles to stabilize your upper body. Too low a back might leave you unnecessarily fatigued from having to balance yourself rather than allowing the chair back to carry you.

At the same time, lower chair backs have become popular, partly as an image issue because they lessen the presence of the wheelchair. A lower back also allows you to rotate more freely, with your shoulders unobstructed. While this is an advantage for those with sufficient balance, it can encourage you in the habit of twisting your body and extending your arms to reach, rather than turning your chair. Over time, such a habit will strain your back, shoulders, and neck.

Many current wheelchair designs allow the vertical support rails of the back of the chair to be set at various heights so that back height can be customized. The upholstery has the ability to adapt to the support heights, with any extra material folding back underneath or running along the seat pan beneath the cushion. It is then held in place with Velcro.

When you order your chair, you will usually specify a back height, which is then adjustable within a range of a few inches.

Back angle

Folding manual chairs usually have an absolutely upright, vertical back because the support rails are part of the entire frame. On fixed-frame designs, the back is able to fold forward for storage of the chair, and so it is mechanically possible for the back angle to be adjustable.

The very act of wheeling typically presses your weight against the back of the chair, just as when a car accelerates you are pressed against your seat. You get better support from a more upright back, so a reclined seat back angle is not necessary for the act of wheeling. What counts is that you feel stable in the chair while sitting normally, allowing the back to carry some of your weight so you don't have to work your trunk muscles unnecessarily.

Leaning back too far in your chair makes it more difficult to push a manual chair, particularly up an incline. Bringing the weight of your upper body into the push helps propel your wheels without having to do all of the work with your arms and shoulders. You'll discover that having something in your lap such as a shopping bag will obstruct the forward movement of your body, making it harder to wheel over the crown of streets, curb cuts, or ramps in your home.

If you are less flexible in the hips, a more reclined position might be necessary, although you should discuss with your physical therapist whether you can increase your flexibility through stretching. If you can't perform such exercises yourself, you can seek the help of a family member, friend, or personal assistant.

If you need to be able to alternate between a reclined and upright position, see Chapter 13.

Push handles

You don't have to include push handles on your chair, but there are some good reasons why you might choose to use them.

If you need to be carried up and down stairs, push handles are important. The horizontal bar commonly seen on rigid chairs is not meant to be used to carry you on stairs. The bar is placed too low for your carriers to lift you with stability; they would have to crouch too low to grip it. Making it easy for others to lift you when necessary is also a consideration when choosing the height of your back—if you choose a lower back, the push handles will also be lower. As with the horizontal bar, carriers won't be able to lift you with stability.

Those with upper-body balance limitations can use the push handles to support themselves when they lean forward to reach. If you aren't able to use the muscles that hold the upper body erect, any forward motion will make the body want to fall the rest of the way. When you reach across the table for the salt or across your desk for the telephone, you need to support yourself with your free arm. The push handle can be a valuable tool for functional stability when you hook your free arm around it.

You can see that push handles might come in handy even if no one ever actually pushes you. You do not have to surrender your independence because your chair is equipped with push handles.

CHAPTER ELEVEN

Footrests

SUPPORTING THE FEET wherever they need to be is very important. One of the risks of using a wheelchair—particularly for power chair users—is to have your foot fall off a footrest, or be improperly supported to begin with, and then be injured by getting caught on an object or literally run over by the chair itself.

Footrests can be stationary or able to move out of the way. Feet might be supported by individual footplates or rest together on a single plate. Feet can be held on the footplates by heel loops or calf supports. The angle of the footrest hangers might be tight, so that the lower legs are perpendicular to the ground, or wider, so that the legs are in a more forward position.

This chapter explains the two kinds of footrests, as well as other associated options, and points out the importance of choosing the best footrest angle for your needs.

Fixed or swingaway?

There are essentially two types of footrests—fixed and swingaway.

Fixed footrests are increasingly common, spurred by the growth and popularity of rigid-frame wheelchairs. They are integrated into the frame of the chair, held in place by telescoping tubes which slide into the frame to be adjusted for your leg length.

A fixed footrest typically has a single metal plate which holds both feet, rather than a separate plate for each foot. The single footplate attaches either between two tubes which extend from the frame or is clamped onto a tube which is part of the frame itself. The single footplate is therefore a design that can add to the structural rigidity of the chair.

And since it involves fewer moving parts, there is less maintenance risk. For an example of a fixed footrest, see Figure 2, "A lightweight, rigid-frame manual wheelchair," in Chapter 7, *Manual Chair Decisions*.

Swingaway footrests are the historical norm and remain an option for some folding wheelchairs. Individual footplates are attached to the bottom of hangers—metal tubes that attach onto the frame structure. A spring release allows the hanger/footrest mechanism to be held in place but easily released to swing the whole unit aside or remove it completely. The ability to remove your footrests can help when sitting at a table with a large base, getting into a very small elevator, approaching a bathtub, or putting your chair into an automobile trunk. For an example of swingaway footrests, see Figure 3, "A lightweight folding manual wheelchair," in Chapter 7. The footplates of swingaway footrests usually flip up to help you transfer to or from the chair. Flip-up plates are mandatory for folding chairs, or the chair would be prevented from closing. (If someone else will be folding your chair, be sure they know the footplates have to be lifted first, to avoid damage to your chair.) Some folding chairs offer the option of a full-width plate, which can also flip up as a single unit to allow the chair to fold. The single plate offers added structural stability as well as more freedom for the positions of your feet.

As you wheel, your feet are kept from sliding off the footplates by heel loops—strips of sturdy material attached and looped across the rear of the footrests. Instead of heel loops, some chairs—usually rigid-frame chairs with single footplates—use a support strap that passes across the frame behind the calves, keeping your feet in place by preventing your legs from sliding backward. Some people find their feet are less stable with a calf-support strap, particularly if they have a tight hanger angle. Feet can more easily slide off the footplate, although tipping the footplate at more of an angle can help.

Angle and position of footrests

The angle of your footrest determines where your feet will be in relation to your knees. A tight angle will put feet under the knees. Some footrests even angle backward, so that feet are farther back than the knees. A wider angle, of course, will bring feet forward so they are in front of the knees. Which angle is best for you depends on a variety of factors, including leg length, physical limitations, and personal preference. In addition to the angle of the footrest, you might also want to consider footrest designs that keep your feet closer together. Finally, consider the best angle for your feet as they rest on the footplate.

Recent designs have brought the angle of the footrests closer to the body, putting the legs into more of a perpendicular position. Table legs become less of an obstacle, removing the need for flip-up footplates for some people. A tighter footrest angle means a shorter "wheelbase" from rear to toe, and so allows you to turn around in smaller spaces. You need sufficient range of motion to bend at the knees and ankles to use these closer footrest angles.

Some people like to be able to see their toes so they can tell where their feet are. If you are conscious of your posture and concerned about your feet being even and flat on the plates, you might want to choose a more forward angle. Those with longer legs might need a more forward angle in order to bring the feet up away from the ground. This option might be more convenient for them than choosing a taller seat height, which can raise the knees too high to clear desks or tables.

For people with flexion contracture, where the knee will not open to a ninety degree angle, the feet need to be supported underneath the leg. Some chair producers have an optional footrest that can be adjusted back underneath the chair. This is generally available only for manual chairs, since batteries and motors usually take up this space.

Another recent trend has been to bring the feet closer together, which helps to reduce the knock-kneed posture that is common for many chair riders. A tapered design, where the footrest hangers angle inward, narrows the profile of the chair at your legs, which can help in passing through tight spaces. A folding chair with tapered footrest hangers will not close completely, stopped by the footplates, which are closer to each other. You might find this type of chair more difficult to load into the car, although once you have opened and closed it enough, it will loosen up and fold to a narrower dimension than when it was new.

The angle of the footplate itself can be either fixed or adjustable, raising or lowering your toes relative to your heels. The more forward the angle of the hanger, the more upward an angle the plate needs to be at to accommodate the natural posture of your feet. Most manufacturers offer an adjustable footplate as an option. This is especially useful for people whose feet are different, who go through changes with contractures in the legs, or who have progressive conditions that affect foot angle.

Be sure the dimensions of your chair include sufficient ground clearance for footrests. ANSI/RESNA recommends two inches of clearance from the ground, but this depends on what sort of terrain you travel, and whether you wheel down steep ramps where the feet need to be higher when you reach the bottom to prevent the footplates from scraping the pavement. If the footrests hit the pavement, your forward movement could be halted abruptly, throwing you from the chair.

Removing footrests

As discussed earlier in this chapter, there may be times when you will need to remove one or both of your footrests. Given the inconvenience of having to remove and reattach your footrests, you might be tempted to leave the footrests off altogether, particularly if you have the use of your legs. But having your feet and legs properly supported has a big effect on the pressures in your spine, excessive forces along the bottom of your thighs against the cushion, and your ability to achieve a natural and relaxed posture—and helps keep you from falling out of the chair! Footrests are important, and if you have a particular access problem that leads you to want to take them off, you are much better off trying to solve the access problem. If that isn't possible, consider the time and effort you spend taking off and putting on your footrests as a worthwhile investment in long-term good health.

CHAPTER TWELVE

Tires, Casters, and Suspension Systems

THE COMFORT OF YOUR RIDE and how well you are able to surmount obstacles in your path are strongly influenced by the tires and casters on your wheelchair, and whether or not it includes a suspension system. It is important that you understand what kinds of tires, casters, and suspension systems are available, and the advantages and disadvantages of each option.

This chapter describes the various kinds of tires and casters, and takes a look at anti-tippers. It also discusses relatively new wheelchair designs that include suspension, and how this feature affects your ride.

Tires

Tires influence the comfort of your ride and the amount of maintenance your chair will need. Some riders also consider the choice of tires an important aesthetic consideration. Generally, wheelchair tires are made of a gray rubber designed not to leave scuff marks on floors. You are unlikely to find them in your local bicycle shop, although the shop might be willing to special-order them for you. Your choices range from pneumatic—air-filled—tires to solid rubber tires, with tires that attempt to offer the best of both in between. As you decide which type of tire will serve you best, keep in mind that larger tires will add width to your chair.

Pneumatic tires have inflatable tubes in them like bicycle tires do, so they offer a more cushioned ride and are better able to squeeze their way over obstacles. Like bicycle tires, they can be punctured by a tack or piece of glass picked up on the street. The risk of punctures is greater for power chair tires because the extra weight of the chair against the pavement can help a sharp object pierce the rubber. Obviously, getting a flat tire means you might find yourself stranded someplace away from home or going back for a repair riding on the deflated tire. Riding on a flat tire can cause damage to the rim of the wheel. Flats can be minimized by using heavy-duty, thorn-resistant tubes or Kevlar tires. (Kevlar is a material used for bulletproof vests.)

Pneumatic tires need replacement more often, since the depth of the rubber before reaching the fiber lining is thinner than a solid tire. The rubber wears down from normal use, particularly the more shallow treads of most manual chair tires. Knobby tires with a deeper tread are also available. They will last longer and provide better traction on unpaved surfaces, but are harder on the hands of manual chair riders.

Thin-profile pneumatic tires—used on manual chairs—have less surface area in contact with the pavement, so there is less friction when turning. This makes the chair more agile, critical for sport use, and preferred by some riders for daily use. Others find the thin-profile tires less comfortable in their hands.

Solid rubber tires make for a rougher ride. You will feel each bump of the pavement, but your tires will never go flat. You might value the security of knowing you will not get a flat, like this power chair user:

> I found when I had air tires on my chair I would get flats an average of two to three times a month. It happened at very inopportune times, like when I was alone or on vacation. Switching to solid tires has been a godsend. Now I don't have to avoid that broken glass. I can go right through it.

Many power chairs have solid tires with a deeper tread that lasts longer while providing better traction. Solid rubber tires tend to be slightly heavier than other options, since they contain more rubber.

A recent variation that is a compromise between pneumatic and solid rubber tires uses a rubber insert. The insert is placed inside a tire as an alternative to an inflatable tube. The tire doesn't need to be pumped up with air, so obviously can't go flat. Manual chair riders will find that the resulting apparent tire pressure is softer and that the chair won't roll as easily. The wheels will also lose momentum faster, which means having to push more often. However, some power chair users swear by rubber inserts.

Yet another variation is the foam-filled tire, a special design that has better rollability and a softer ride, but cannot go flat.

Casters

Casters are the smaller wheels at the front (usually) of your wheelchair that allow the chair to turn—and keep it from tipping over on two wheels. Casters rotate on their forks as you change direction in your chair. They can be large or small, soft or hard. The kind of casters you choose has a lot of impact on your comfort and mobility. You will want to weigh the advantages of small casters against those of large casters.

Small casters allow tighter footrest angles, thus their popularity on rigid-frame chairs. Small casters are less likely to get in a position that prevents them from rotating when you turn. Greater agility has made small casters very popular, but since they are hard—typically made of solid plastic or rubber—they make for a bumpier ride. Some small caster wheels are the same type as those used on rollerblades or skateboards. You will feel every crack in the sidewalk, and you will need to lift the casters by doing a mini-wheelie with an extra push in order to clear thresholds at doorways. The smallest types of casters can even be stopped by very small obstacles, like a stone on a sidewalk. They might get caught in a sewer or ventilation grate on the street. These kinds of sudden stops, as you know, can mean being thrown out of your chair.

Pneumatic casters are larger, at least six inches in diameter. They will provide a very soft ride. Any air-filled tire is at risk of puncture, but it is also true that a flat caster will not strand you the way a flat main tire will. The chair itself will also last longer with larger, soft casters, as the vibration from harder tires causes more wear and tear on the frame.

Large casters can handle obstacles and rough terrain more easily. Picture a hard caster approaching a three-inch curb, and you can sense that it would require more force to roll over the curb than a softer, larger tire would. The TerraTrek all-terrain chair from Kuschall has very large, pneumatic front casters, partnered with heavy-duty knobby main tires.

Before choosing a large caster, you'll want to consider your ideal footrest angle. When larger, pneumatic casters are used, your heels must be moved forward with a greater footrest angle to clear the rotation of the casters, extending your overall length, "wheel to toe," if you will.

Larger casters can also obstruct your movement suddenly if you are close to a wall or some other raised surface. As the caster begins to rotate, it becomes blocked by the wall, stopping your movement. You won't be trapped; you'll simply have to maneuver so that you get the caster free of the obstacle. Some people find this stressful, but many users learn to avoid these situations.

A compromise between the two extremes of caster options is the four-inch solid rubber caster. It cannot be punctured, is not stopped by small obstacles, but does still transmit more vibration through the chair.

Comparison of Tire Types for Wheels and Casters

Type of tire	Advantages	Disadvantages
Pneumatic (air-filled)	Cushioned ride. Surmounts obstacles more easily. Less wear and tear.	Can be punctured. Needs replacement more often. On casters, does not allow tight footrest angle.on chair frame. Makes chair less agile.
Solid rubber	Won't go flat. On casters, allows tighter footrest angle. Gives chair more agility.	Rougher ride. Slightly heavier.
Rubber insert	Won't go flat. Works well on power chairs.	Requires more energy to push manual chair.
Foam-filled	Won't go flat. Softer ride. Easier to push than rubber insert.	Doesn't last as long.

Anti-tippers

You should always err on the side of safety, so consider using the anti-tippers many chairs offer as an option. Small wheels are attached to the end of a metal arm that slides into the bottom frame tube at the rear of the chair. The wheels float a couple of inches off the ground, so that if you tip back you will be kept from falling.

Sometimes the anti-tippers can be used as rear wheels to get your wheelchair through the narrow aisle of an airplane, once your main wheels have been removed using quick-release axles.

At the end of a steep ramp or when going over a moderate curb, the anti-tippers could cause your main wheels to be lifted off the ground, trapping you on the anti-tippers and front casters. Most designs can be flipped up to temporarily disable the tipping protection so you can be carried up stairs or down a steeper ramp.

Scooters and some power chairs have small wheels integrated into the rear of the frame or modular base, which perform an anti-tipping role. They may or may not be adjustable.

Suspensions

Cars have shock absorbers to soften the ride, so why not wheelchairs? This thought is occurring to an increasing number of chair designers. Outdoor terrain and vibrations from wheeling on sidewalks with all of their bumps and potholes have an impact on the tissues of the body. It is not good for us to be shaken up every day, so a soft ride is protective for people who encounter lots of vibration when they wheel. If you have back discomfort that is aggravated by the bounce of your wheelchair, adding a suspension system can reduce the impact enough to spare you some back pain.

The point of four-wheel independent suspension in a car is not just a soft ride. It is also to maintain optimal traction and control. If one wheel hits a change in surface, it can rise or lower separately from the others. This way, all wheels stay in contact with the ground.

As we've already discussed, one concern about rigid-frame chairs is that they are less able to keep all four wheels in contact with surfaces that are not level, such as an outdoor trail or a city sidewalk with bumps and dips. This instability can mean a temporary loss of control, which potentially could be disastrous. Independent suspension designs enable rigid-frame chairs to have better contact with the ground.

The first commercial chair to appear with four-wheel independent suspension was the Iron Horse, a heavy-duty, folding manual chair. The Iron Horse chair features independent suspension at all four wheels and is advertised as "a chair that softens the hardest terrain." Rear suspension is a key feature of the Boing chair from Colours of Permobil. The Boing chair is a lightweight, rigid-frame chair. Although the Boing is a fixed-frame chair, some of the energy of your push is lost to the suspension, akin to the concern of losing power to a folding frame.

Everest & Jennings have also joined the suspension fray with their Barracuda manual chair and the Lancer power chair. The Invacare Action Storm power chairs all include independent suspension as a standard feature.

Smaller power chair producers have shown a lot of interest in suspension. Power chairs that offer suspension in the design include the OmegaTrac from Teftec and the HiRider from Falcon Rehabilitation Products. The OmegaTrac was designed specifically to handle changes in terrain and to provide confident driving over roots and rocks and dips in unpaved environments. Their drive system is engineered to minimize the impact on straight steering and consistent speed. The HiRider—also a sitting/standing chair—is able to use smaller wheels, thanks to the suspension. Smaller wheels means that the profile of the whole chair is narrower.

A third-party product of interest is called Frog Legs. Frog Legs are a set of casters that have suspension springs built into the forks to soften your ride. The manufacturer claims they reduce vibration and help you hop (thus the name) over obstacles.

CHAPTER THIRTEEN

Tilt/Recline Systems and Positioning Systems

IN ADDITION TO THE VARIETY OF OPTIONS for a basic chair, there are additional features available if your physical condition requires more support, alternative methods for pressure relief, or the ability to shift to a more horizontal position. Your doctor or therapist will no doubt recommend such features if your upper-body balance and stability are seriously limited; your disability involves structural deformities, spinal curvature, or muscle contracture; you are at risk

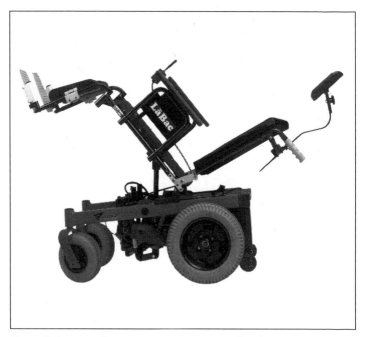

Figure 9. A power tilt seating system on a power drive base

of fainting or dysreflexia; or if you do not have the strength to shift your position on your own.

This chapter will explain the difference between tilting and reclining, and will discuss various issues to consider when choosing a tilt or recline system. Lateral and head supports are also discussed.

Tilt and recline

Chair riders need to have some strategy for shifting the pressure on their spine, sit bones, and skin surfaces. For people with very limited strength or deformities that make it posturally difficult for them to lift themselves, a tilt or recline mechanism—available on both manual and power chairs—might be the answer.

Although similar, tilt and recline are two separate features. When equipped with the tilt feature, the entire seat assembly of the chair tips backward, seat and footrests included. (See Figure 9, "A power tilt

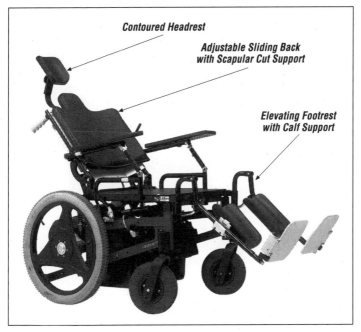

Figure 10. A power chair with recline system

seating system on a power drive base.") The recline feature allows the back of the wheelchair to angle backward, independent of the rest of the chair. (See Figure 10, "A power chair with recline system.")

With a tilt system, the legs will naturally come up as the whole chair tilts backward. But with a recline system, it may or may not be desirable for the legs to rise. It is typical to have elevating footrests on a reclining chair, since when you bend backward at the hips, ligaments and muscles that travel down into your legs are put in tension, wanting to pull your legs up. This is especially true to the degree that you have muscle contractures that prevent your knees from lying flat when you lie down. Some controls will automatically elevate the legs as you recline, but these can also be separate functions.

Generally, tilt and recline chairs use a taller back than chairs without these features, since your upper back requires support when you recline beyond a certain angle. With either feature, a headrest is usually necessary for the times when you are tipped back.

When you are in a reclined position with either of these features, the physical forces on your vertebrae are reduced since your weight is no longer pressing vertically down on your spine. Pressure on the sit bones is reduced considerably. The weight of your body is being transferred to the back of the chair. Less of your weight is transferred to your seat, so pressures change across the skin surfaces in contact with the cushion. Circulation is helped. And it is just a plain relief to have a change in position.

In some cases, both tilt and recline features might be incorporated into the chair. Using tilt first helps maintain posture, but some additional reclining relative to the seat might still be necessary to accomplish sufficient pressure relief. Your therapist will be able to determine if you need a combination of tilt and recline.

If you require a fixed recline angle that you use at all times, select a chair with a back that can be set to your exact needs, but would rarely need to be changed. See the section "Back angle" in Chapter

10, *Seats and Backs*.

Tilt and recline systems are generally motorized, controlled by a switch that is sometimes integrated into the same control box used to drive a power chair. The control switch can also be in a separate location. The electronic equipment that actuates tilt and recline systems is located either underneath the seat or behind the back. Either location has advantages and disadvantages.

Placing the actuator under the seat is the most stable because the weight of the equipment is kept low and toward the center of gravity. This location is usually necessary when the chair includes a portable ventilator, which is placed on a tray behind the seat back. (A back-mounted actuator would bump into the vent and obstruct the recline angle.) The disadvantage of placing the tilt or recline actuator under the seat is that it can increase the seat-to-floor height of the chair.

When seat-to-floor height needs to be kept low, locating the actuator on the back frees space under the seat. However, a back-mounted actuator is more likely to cause the chair to tip backward. The actuator and its mounting hardware are heavy. Remember that the footrests also come up during recline, shifting the center of gravity farther—however slightly—toward the rear of the chair. A longer wheel base is usually required to ensure stability.

It should be possible to defeat the drive control of a power chair while in the tilt/recline position. It can be safe to drive while in a slightly reclined position, so some chairs allow you to define an angle at which driving will not be possible.

Tilt and recline systems from companies such as LaBac, TiltMaster, and Falcon are designed to be used with power chairs from major suppliers like Quickie, Everest & Jennings, and Invacare. Since your chair may consist of components from different manufacturers, it is especially important for your therapist and dealer to make sure you are specifying compatible systems.

Large chair makers like Permobil and Invacare also offer tilt and recline systems of their own, or are expanding into tilt and recline products through acquisition. TiltMaster has been purchased by Sunrise Medical, which owns the Quickie line. Graham-Field, which owns Everest & Jennings, has purchased LaBac. Hopefully, the integration of tilt and recline mechanisms with chair manufacturing will translate into shared engineering and design, which will produce better integration and more variety of choice.

Minimizing shear with recline systems

Shear is horizontal force along the surface of your skin. When only your chair back reclines, there is a tendency for your body to slide forward in the seat. This pressure—shear—is a risk factor for skin breakdown.

As you return to sitting upright, you will probably not be in the same position on the seat cushion as you were before you reclined. Most likely, you will be somewhat slumped in the seat. At worst, the inevitable slumping will increase the risk of spinal deformity. At best, it will be uncomfortable. The more frequently you recline throughout the day, the more significant this issue will be for you.

Producers of recline systems have tried to address the problem of shear and position changes. LaBac (pronounced lay-back), perhaps the largest maker of tilt and recline systems, offers an "adjustable sliding back" that moves with you as the back reclines. Falcon Rehabilitation's system allows the seat to move instead. Each approach is an attempt to allow many reclines while preserving your position when you return to sitting upright. Jeff Ewing of Falcon claims:

> With our recline system, the seat moves, so you can recline back as many as twenty times, and you'll still be in the same position when you come back up. Your hips will still be all the way back in the chair.

Karl Ylonen of Care Corporation has been selling wheelchairs and tilt systems for more than ten years. Ylonen asserts:

> With just a recline system, I don't care who it's from, there is some displacement and some shear going on.

The phrase "zero shear" was once used by companies like LaBac, but not anymore. Zero shear is impossible. The best they can do is reduce it.

If you do not have the upper-body strength to reposition yourself after returning from a reclined posture, you might need to use a tilt system instead. Tilt would also be better if you aren't able to bend comfortably at the hips. Since tilt moves the seat and footrests with the seat back, your entire relationship to the chair remains constant. There is also less weight on your sitting bones, although you must take care not to create excessive sacral pressure, as this is a bony area that is also at high risk of skin breakdown.

Lateral supports

Many people using power chairs—or manual chairs with assistance—have significantly limited upper-body balance or no use of trunk muscles at all. These riders may require the use of lateral supports to keep the upper body in a stable posture.

For simple lateral support, you might choose one of the increasing number of back cushions that are contoured. (See Figure 8, "A deep contour back," in Chapter 10, Seats and Backs.) These back cushions wrap slightly around you to provide some lateral support when the centrifugal force of turning your chair—perhaps too fast!—pushes you to the side.

The less you are able to use your trunk muscles, the more you will need additional lateral supports. The curved shape of a seat back will not be sufficient. Pads mounted on chair arms and attached to either side of the chair come in various sizes, shapes, and thicknesses, depending on your need. Lateral supports may be removable and/or may swing away for ease of transfer. Some riders will use these pads for support only when they need it, such as while driving the chair. Others, such as high-level quadriplegic riders, whose upper-body stability is precarious, need to be actually held in place by supports.

There is also a psychological component to having supports. Karl Ylonen of Care Corporation points out:

> A lot of people have a fear of falling sideways or forward. The more snug you get them in their chair, the more comfortable and secure they will feel.

If you are to be in continual contact with lateral supports, your therapist and dealer must take great care to choose the right pads. There is a risk of pressure sores from too small and too firm a pad pressing against your sides, made even more dangerous if you are not able to sense the pad. You might need to take breaks from being in your chair during the day in order to minimize the risk of pressure sores. You certainly will need to give extra attention to the care and inspection of those areas of your skin that come into contact with support pads.

Some riders prefer an approach for maintaining stability that is less complicated, less risky to skin surfaces, and cheaper. While in their chair they simply use a seat belt across their chest.

Head support

As with lateral support, some people require constant stabilization of their head. Others rely on head support only when using a tilt or recline system. Headrests come in many shapes and designs.

Headrests are often one of the most difficult pieces of the puzzle to fit into the choosing of a chair. Muscle tone and range of the neck have to be considered. Sometimes the best position for the head in terms of muscle strength and position is not the same as where the head needs to be for optimal vision. You also have to take care not to risk pressure sores from continual contact with a headrest.

Getting the headrest into the right position can be a challenge. People who use headrests generally also require the support of a tall seat back. Getting the head support in just the right place so it is comfortable and safe can be difficult with all of the hardware and upholstery in the area.

If you require head support, be sure to get expert help in choosing the right design and having it placed correctly. Take your time to ensure the best support and most comfort, with minimal inconvenience.

CHAPTER FOURTEEN

Armrests, Clothing Guards, and Accessories

ARMRESTS OFFER SUPPORT AND STABILITY and allow you to shift your position more easily. They can also get in the way when you are sitting at a desk or when you're wheeling your manual chair. What type of armrests you choose, or whether you choose not to have them, depends on a variety of factors, including your upper-body balance, your lifestyle, and your particular needs.

Clothing guards are another optional feature, often included as part of the armrests. Clothing guards protect your clothes from coming into contact with the wheels of the chair. In some cases, they also help hold the seat cushion in place and prevent the wheels from rubbing against it.

This chapter discusses the pros and cons of armrests for those who have a choice, as well as some of the various types of armrests available. Clothing guard options are also discussed. Finally, this chapter includes a brief review of some of the many accessories available for riders.

Do you need armrests?

Power chairs almost always have armrests, but some manual chair riders feel that armrests get in their way. It's true that armrests can interfere with wheeling when you want to get your body into the push by leaning forward, and people with shorter arms in particular might find that armrests interfere with a comfortable relationship to the wheels. Armrests can also get in the way of reaching to the side or to the floor, or prevent you from being able to get close enough to a table at work or in a restaurant. In addition, armrests add weight to the chair—a significant amount in some cases.

But before you decide against armrests for your manual chair, consider the following benefits of having them:

- Armrests can help prevent spinal problems. Sitting puts pressure on the spine, and the weight of your arms and shoulder girdle adds to that pressure. Researchers suspect that over the long term, a wheelchair user might develop problems in the discs of the spine, which can cause compression of nerves passing between the vertebrae. When you put the weight of your arms on armrests, you relieve some of the load on your spine.

- Armrests may be important for transfers into and out of the chair.

- Armrests are helpful for shifting your weight in the chair, a crucial habit for the prevention of pressure sores. Although some people are able to do their push-ups without armrests—using the wheels or bracing their palms on their cushion—you can lift yourself higher using armrests, helping the circulation in your legs.

- If you have limited upper-body balance, your safety may depend on having armrests. The act of wheeling the chair subjects your body to forces that can cast you out of your wheels; armrests offer a source of stability. Then there are those times when you are reaching for something or are on an inclined surface, which can lead to a sudden fall if you are not taking extra care in the way you move. Falls can also happen when you are being pushed in the chair, as the person pushing you might not be sensitive to the subtle shifts in balance you experience while in motion. To the degree that balance is an issue for you, having armrests can make the difference between staying in the chair or getting a close look at the pavement.

Generally, armrests are removable, so nothing says that you have to use them all the time. Many chair users purchase armrests, and then use them only when it is appropriate for them.

> *My habit is to get dressed while sitting in my chair, and I rely on armrests to lift myself high enough to pull up my pants. More recently I've been spending more time at the computer and find that armrests offer some relief to my neck and shoulders. Otherwise, I leave them off.*

As always, the choice depends on your individual needs and activities.

Types of armrests

There are several types of armrests. The typical armrest is wide enough to support the arm, is padded, and is covered with vinyl upholstery. This type of armrest can be in the desk style—which has a shorter upholstered section, allowing you to pull closer to desks and tables—or full-length, which might be important to support a lap tray if you use one.

Some armrests lock down and can be used as a grip to carry a folded chair or used by people who might carry you on a stairway. If the armrests on your chair are not fixed, be certain to let someone helping you know this before they attempt to lift your chair—especially if you are in it. Locking arms also ensure that the armrests will still be with the chair when you reclaim it after an airline trip.

High-level quadriplegic riders can choose sculpted armrests, possibly with straps, to keep their arms in place. Some riders may have enough dexterity to operate a joystick control on a power chair, even though their arms are generally weak. Sculpted armrests can aid them in keeping their arms in place while driving the chair. Sculpted armrests might also include supports for the hands and fingers to keep them from curling into contracture.

Many modern manual chairs have tube-design, swingaway armrests that can easily rotate away from the chair. The horizontal portion is covered with a soft, water-resistant material. These armrests tend not to be comfortable for resting your arms, because they are round and not very wide. Tube-design armrests are more appropriate for doing push-ups and correcting yourself if you feel off-balance.

There are also flip-up armrests, a good solution for those who need/want armrests only part of the time, but who don't want the bother of taking them off and putting them back on.

Whatever type of armrests you choose, it is important to adjust them to the correct height. Armrests that are too high will lead you to elevate your shoulders, which can cause tight muscles and pain in the neck and shoulders. If armrests are too low, you will be encouraged to slump to the side to make contact, increasing the risk of developing spinal curvature.

Your armrests can be height-adjustable in one of several ways. Some designs use a telescoping support that you can change at any time. For instance, you might find it desirable to raise the height of armrests for transfers and lower them out of the way while wheeling. Other chairs provide several fixed positions, where the bolts that support the armrest are installed when the chair is configured. Be certain that the person who assembles your chair accounts properly for the position of your arms.

Clothing guards

Clothing guards—also called sideguards—protect clothes from being soiled by or getting caught in the wheels of the chair. They are optional, but if you will be riding your chair outside very much, clothing guards are a practical choice. You can select armrests with built-in clothing guards. Those who do not use armrests, or who prefer the tubular type, which includes no side panel, can use separate sideguards. Clothing guards can be made of fabric, plastic, or metal.

Wheels pick up dirt—and other substances—from the ground. Imagine a farm or a city street where lots of pets are walked. Chair riders need to watch where they are wheeling. (Manual chair riders need to be especially cautious lest they find their hands soiled in some unfortunate way.) Even when you are careful, dirt from the wheels can get on your clothes, although this is less likely if you have a power chair with smaller wheels.

If you are wearing a long coat or dress, there is a risk of it getting caught in the works. Many armrests include side panels that keep clothes contained within the seat and protect your slacks or skirt. If you do not have armrests, you will want to consider whether fabric or rigid clothing guards will best suit your needs.

The advantages of using cloth sideguards are that they are lightweight and can be easily loosened when you need to move them out of the way, during transfers, for instance.

The disadvantages are that the flexibility of cloth sideguards makes them tend to bend outward from general use. When this happens, your clothing will not be completely contained. Cloth sideguards are typically held in place by a cord that attaches to an eyelet on the back of the chair. With time and usage, the eyelet can pull off, requiring the replacement of the back. Cloth sideguards must be adjusted often to maintain the tension necessary to pull the cloth up into position. These constant adjustments can be aggravating. If you don't keep the guards in the proper position, the wheels might rub against them as you move, making an irritating sound and leaving a track of dirt. Finally, in order to take off cloth sideguards, you must take the sling seat off of the chair, first removing, then replacing the bolts that hold the seat in place.

In contrast, plastic sideguards are rigid, and are held on by a thin bar that inserts into a slot mounted on the chair frame. They can be removed by being lifted out of the slot. (If you remove and replace them often, a bit of oil to keep them lubricated might be necessary.) Since plastic sideguards do not get crushed down as the cloth ones do, they are more effective in holding in your clothing.

The main disadvantage of plastic sideguards is that they require extra care during transfers. You can injure your skin by hitting the hard edge, potentially causing a sore. You might also break the sideguard. Finally, plastic guards can be an obstruction if you sometimes sit cross-legged in your wheelchair.

Accessories

Most wheelchair manufacturers—certainly the large ones—also offer an array of accessories to go along with your wheels. Invacare will embroider your name on the seat back. You can order such things as holders for crutches or for a cup of coffee. For shopping, there are products such as the Front Runner, a carrying basket that sits on two supports that fold down from the footrest hangers. There are lap trays, book holders, weather canopies, and all sorts of pouches and bags.

The ideal pouch is pretty important. When seated, it's harder to take advantage of pockets in pants or coats. But it's still necessary to have someplace to put wallets, keys, books, or business materials. Briefcases don't work very well, since they just slide off your lap as you ride, unless you want to fuss with bungie cords to strap them down. A pouch might also be needed for medications or catheterization supplies, which are standard cargo for many wheelers.

I have a beloved leather bag that was modified with a couple of loops so it could hang off the push handles of my chair. It's been a trusted companion since 1974, and even survived the attack of a stray dog on the street. And it looks its age. Having made the switch to a rigid frame, I've bought a bag that attaches beneath the seat, with plenty of zippered pockets and secure storage. It even improves the center of gravity a bit, especially if I need to tip back for a wheelie or go up a ramp.

More dexterity and balance are needed to reach a bag under the seat, so many people opt for one that hangs on the back of the chair. Even that requires you to twist around to reach behind you while remaining stable. (Be sure to switch directions rather than always turning the same way—this will help prevent a chronic twist in your spine over the long term.) A bag hanging on the back of your chair might interfere with making adjustments to an adjustable support back, or, with a deep back, might protrude too far out from the chair and bump into things when you turn. On the other hand, a back-mounted bag can be useful for an attendant who accompanies you on an outing or meets you at a place of employment to briefly help with some task.

If placing your bag under or in back of the seat isn't manageable, or if you usually travel light, the easiest, although smallest, solution is a pack that hangs off the side of an armrest.

CHAPTER FIFTEEN

Wheelchair Maintenance

LIKE ANYTHING ELSE OF VALUE that you own and use regularly, your wheelchair will last much longer and serve you better if you take good care of it. A little bit of regular, preventive maintenance will make a big difference in the performance and endurance of your wheels. The manual that comes with your wheelchair will discuss maintenance. Your dealer should also be happy to talk with you about maintenance and can set up dates to have your chair checked.

You, or someone assisting you, can do many of the more common preventive maintenance tasks yourself, and if you have a way with fixing things, you might be able to handle most of the maintenance on a manual wheelchair. Most wheelchair makers offer a toolkit as an accessory. It typically includes the wrenches, screwdrivers, or other tools to adjust all of the nuts, bolts, and screws on your chair. Such a toolkit can be especially handy if you travel.

Power chairs are another story. They are quite complex and need the attention of a skilled technician. Even so, there are measures you can take on your own to extend the life and quality of a power chair.

This chapter will tell you the essentials of good wheelchair maintenance and offer tips about what to look for to avoid problems.

Keep your chair clean

Dirt and grime get into small places where moving parts can be worn down. A dirty chair will age faster, so it is important to clean your chair regularly. If you are outside a lot, you'll probably want to clean your chair every week—perhaps more often if you frequently ride over unpaved terrain.

Your chair can be kept generally clean with a cloth and gentle cleanser. Avoid abrasive cloths and sponges—particularly steel wool—that can scratch surfaces. Also avoid petroleum-based cleaners, which can be damaging to your upholstery. You might want to consider environment-friendly cleansers that will not only respect your local water supply, but also spare you from exposure to unnecessarily strong chemicals.

As you tour around your chair while cleaning, watch for these details:

- Are there cracks in any vinyl upholstery? Exposed cracks can be a source of skin irritation.

- Are there scratches in the finish of the frame? The manufacturer probably can sell you a bottle of touch-up paint, even for glitter finishes.

- Many earlier wheelchairs still in use have a chrome finish that can peel, leaving a sharp edge that can be quite dangerous if you don't see it. Be on the lookout for these edges to avoid cutting yourself.

- Is the frame tight or does it wobble at its joints? Check screws and bolts to ensure they are tight, particularly at the axle plates, swingaway footrest mechanisms, caster axles, motor and battery housings, and so on. Don't make them too tight, though. You could deform the frame, cause moving parts to become too stiff, or make the screws and bolts difficult to loosen in the future.

- Fibrous material tends to collect in the caster axles since they are so close to the ground. Hairs and threads easily get wrapped around the axle, and the only way to clean them is to remove the caster from the fork. All you need are two wrenches, one to hold the axle bolt in place so it doesn't turn and one to unscrew the nut. There are two small spacers on either side of the caster wheel that you must be careful not to lose. These are where the threads and such collect.

- Are pneumatic tires evenly set on the wheel rims? Tires have a "bead," which is an edge meant to sit inside the rim. You can tell if it is not set consistently, in which case your ride will not be as smooth and the tube could potentially push the tire off the rim. This is particularly a concern for composite wheels, which tend to have less of a lip to receive the bead.

- Is there grease leaking from around the wheel axles or other joints? A small amount might be normal, but more could indicate a loss of lubricant worth your concern. Another indication of lost lubricant would be if your folding chair became more difficult to open or close.

- Check the heel loops on the footrests for worn material. Sometimes the stitching that wraps around the footrest hanger comes apart, so this is a place you should keep an eye on. You might even want to proactively reinforce it with some extra stitching.

Tires, wheels, and casters

You'll want to perform regular checks on your tires, wheels, and casters, in addition to the more general observations you make while cleaning. The frequency of these checks depends on how much, and how strenuously, you use your chair.

- Check your tire pressure. Tires will wear faster if they are not kept at their maximum pressure, which is marked on the side of the tires. Your brakes will also be effectively weakened, since softer tires will make less firm contact. In addition, softer tires make a chair harder to push for manual riders, and use up the batteries faster on a power chair.

  If you are a manual rider, your hands-on contact with your tires every day will allow you to have a sense of when the pressure is low. Power chair tires can be checked with a pressure gauge—every couple of weeks should be adequate, unless you have reason to believe the pressure might be low.

- Spin your wheels. They should turn very easily without any grinding sound. Such a sound indicates damaged bearings that should be replaced.

- Test spoke tension with the wheelchair on its side or the wheels removed, so there is no load on the wheels. (Even the weight of the wheelchair will cause the upper spokes to carry more tension than the lower ones.) The spokes should all have equal tension. One loose spoke will cause the others to carry more tension. Ultimately the wheel will go out of round. Adjusting spoke tension is best done by a qualified technician. Over-tightening some spokes can damage the wheel.

  If spoke tension is unequal, you may hear a faint, metallic, snapping sound as you ride. Even if this symptom isn't present, it's a good idea to check spoke tension about once a month if you're quite active, less frequently if you're not.

- Check the casters and forks about once a month. Casters and forks should rotate freely and smoothly. The caster fork should not wiggle on its axle. If it is loose, the entire caster assembly will shake once it is rolling fast enough, a sign to watch for as you use your chair.

- Do all four wheels touch the floor evenly? If not, there could be a serious problem with the alignment of the chair frame, possibly even a crack or failing weld. If you suspect a problem with the frame, it should be investigated immediately. A small caster that does not touch the ground might only require a simple adjustment of the fork axle or the plate attaching it to the frame. Some chairs allow height adjustment of the caster axle assemblies.

- Check wheel locks to make sure they are firm enough. Wheel locks tend to loosen with use.

Look—and listen—for problems

One of the most important things you can do to avoid costly and inconvenient repairs is to be aware of how your wheelchair looks, sounds, and feels when it is new and properly adjusted. Become familiar with all the parts of the chair so you will be able to spot when something looks different. A properly functioning chair also has its own sounds—or lack of them. If you are attuned to how your chair sounds when it's running smoothly, you will easily notice any inappropriate noise such as a squeaky frame, a grinding axle, or a damaged motor. Finally, be aware of how your wheelchair feels when you are in it. Your chair becomes an extension of your body, and familiarity with it will alert you to something that isn't quite right.

Following are some specific problems to watch for:

- If your chair doesn't wheel consistently straight, or if your folding chair doesn't open and close easily, there might be damage to the frame. Don't ignore these kinds of symptoms if you notice them during normal use of the chair.

- Soft upholstery becomes loose from the stretching it endures over time from your body weight. Chair backs with adjustable straps need regular attention. It is usually easiest to enlist someone's help to tighten these straps since it is awkward to reach behind yourself and pull them tight.

- Sling-seat upholstery also gets loose from your weight. It is important not to allow your seat to sag; this allows your cushion to bend, which could damage it. A seat that is sagging compromises your postural support and optimal protection from pressure sores. Some sling seats can be adjusted by removing one side from the frame and then pulling the material tight before replacing it.

- Keep heel loop studs tight—partly to avoid losing the bolt. The small bolt that goes up through the bottom of the footrest has nothing to hold it in place if it comes out. You might not discover it is gone until your foot slides off the footrest.

    When I was in Paris, I lost one of the bolts that holds my heel loops in place. I had to spend a couple of days constantly adjusting my foot until I found a hardware store on a side street. At least I got to learn how to say "bolt" in French (boulon).

Power wheelchair maintenance

Even if you are unable to perform any of the required maintenance for your power chair, you are still an important part of making sure it stays in top condition. As discussed in the previous section, you can visually observe the parts of your chair, noticing problems that are apparent. For example, observe any moving parts such as belts, gears, and wheels to make sure that wiring is safely away from them with no chance of being caught. It might be necessary to tie wires down to the frame or in a bunch to each other. There are products made to clip wires to another surface to ensure they do not interfere with moving parts.

You can also call attention to anything that doesn't feel the way it normally does, such as a loose armrest. Perhaps most important, you can learn enough about how your chair works, and how parts are connected, to be able to instruct someone so they can fix a minor problem or loose connection.

Listen to your motor. It is a good idea to become familiar with the healthy sound of your wheelchair when it is new. Over time, just like a car, it will become a little noisier, but if your ear is tuned to how it sounds when it is healthy, you will be able to notice when there is excessive noise. Increased noise might indicate worn bearings, out of line belts or gears, or frame problems. Some chairs have a motor for each wheel. Each should sound the same.

In addition to these general observations, you will want to do specific checks on the following:

- If your chair uses drive belts, check them monthly for proper tightness and alignment. If they are loose, they are more likely to fall off or slip, wasting drive power. If they are too tight, they could cause damage to the bearings in the motor and ultimately mean costly repairs.

- Although not required as regularly as some of the other checks, you will need to check electrical connections from time to time to make sure they are firmly in place and are free of grime and corrosion. For instance, you might want to check to make sure all connections are tight after someone else has worked on your chair.

If you live where the winters are harsh and the roads are salted, you will need to clean the electrical connections on your chair more often to protect them from salt corrosion. Buildup can be removed with a wire brush after removing the cable from the connection. (If it will not come off at first, your local hardware store has products, such as Liquid Wrench™, that help to loosen stuck parts.) Apply a small amount of petroleum grease to limit corrosion.

Do not risk any unintentional changes of wiring connections. A good chair design will color-code the wires, and if you remove one you should note its color. In fact, don't remove more than one connection at a time, so that there will be no chance of replacing it in the wrong place. Putting wires back incorrectly is quite dangerous. At the least, you could damage the electrical system of the chair. At worst, you could cause a short-circuit, which could burn you.

- Any moving part that you use a lot, such as footrests, removable backs, tilt mechanisms, or adjustable armrests are likely to wear out sooner than other parts of the chair simply because they get more use.

  The thing I've needed repaired most often is the right armrest, which comes loose and wants to hang down. This is the side where my joystick is located. It happens because of me leaning on armrests to boost myself up or position myself better. My repair guy says it's a design flaw.

CHAPTER SIXTEEN

Wheeling Style and Technique

YOU ARE GOING TO BECOME AN EXPERT at driving your chair. It is the nature of the body to gain coordination simply from the act of doing—the more we perform a particular task, the better our nervous and muscular systems adapt to that task. All of us can remember learning a skill that was awkward at first, whether it was tying our shoes, playing a sport or musical instrument, or cutting vegetables. Even if you have never had the use of your arms, you gained dexterity with your head and mouth, perhaps as a painter or computer operator. This "practice makes perfect" principle is equally true for the skill of driving your wheels.

You will develop a refined sense of how to operate your chair. The push and pull of the wheels or the control of a joystick will become ingrained in you, second nature, as nearly an unconscious act as walking for those who are able.

This chapter discusses what is necessary to achieve optimal wheeling, introduces manual chair riders to the technique of using wheelies to get over obstacles, and explains the advantages of wheeling with mindfulness.

Optimal wheeling

In order for you to become adept at maneuvering your wheelchair, it is important that you have the right chair for you, and that it is properly adjusted for your needs. The wide array of wheelchair products and professional expertise available are intended to provide you with a means of mobility appropriate to your physical ability while allowing you the best possible level of participation in your life's activities. Optimal comfort and ease while riding in your chair are included in that goal. Using your chair should not be fatiguing. After you've had time to get used to your wheelchair, continued awkwardness or difficulty operating the chair may mean that your wheels are not what you need them to be. For instance, a manual chair might be too heavy or be improperly adjusted, or you might have the wrong cushion. Or the difficulties could mean that you should be using a power chair.

When you have the right chair and have learned the basics of getting around in it, time, practice, and experience will lead you to a high level of expertise in making your chair do what you want it to do. But it is style and grace that will distinguish you as a true master of your wheels.

For instance, faster isn't always better. For power chair riders, too much speed can be dangerous, for the obvious reason that you can be thrown from your wheels. Going too fast makes it harder for you to control the chair, as you must brace your body against the various forces and sheer momentum of traveling so fast.

Some manual chair riders waste energy by wheeling faster than necessary. This is an inefficient way to use the body and is more fatiguing than a relaxed style of wheeling, if only because going fast often means that you keep pushing the wheels rather than allowing yourself to coast between pushes. It is easy to imagine that, if you allow brief breaks between pushes, bringing your arms back in an unrushed manner, you will do fewer pushes for the same distance and therefore expend less effort.

Many manual chair riders seem to push with an almost frantic style, wheeling fast, doing their most to demonstrate their dexterity and agility to the outside world:

> *Looking back, I can see clearly how much I was invested in being the hotshot wheelchair rider in the early years of my disability, which*

happened when I was eighteen. Wheeling slowly somehow made me feel more disabled, a purely psychological response to how I imagined the public saw me. Surely, I seemed to think, if they see how agile and strong I am with my wheels, they won't think I'm a "cripple" and everything I imagined to be associated with that image.

It's a mistake to be so concerned with what people are thinking and with what their cultural assumptions might be in regard to disability. It truly doesn't matter what other people think. Of course, saying that what people think doesn't matter is considerably easier than really not caring about it. It's a natural psychological feature of disability to focus on how others perceive us, and it takes a while to break through this barrier.

Putting our awareness on how we appear to others prevents us from putting our awareness on what we're doing. If we are thinking about how we're viewed, we tend to be less focused on where we're going, and are more likely to bump into something, jam a thumb on the brake, or do some just plain klutzy thing in our chairs. It's when we are relaxed and mindful of where we are and what we are doing that we are more graceful and confident as we wheel. We end up looking more competent—able, if you will—to others after all.

By taking your time, you will also reduce the cumulative strain on your shoulders, elbows, and wrists, which can ultimately cost you the ability to use a manual chair later in life. Some people who are aging with disability are losing the ability to push a manual chair for this very reason. Slow down just a bit, and you will exhibit more grace, have more energy for your day, and preserve your independence throughout your lifetime.

You're likely to find that a more relaxed wheeling style doesn't slow you down significantly, and you can certainly still have fun in your wheels:

I have a favorite block in San Francisco with a really wide side-walk. It doesn't slope too steeply toward the street, but has a great downhill slope at a moderate pitch. It's perfect because I can build up some good speed, but not so fast I lose control. Better than most amusement park rides!

Negotiating curbs and obstacles

How well you are able to move over changes in surface levels is affected by how your wheelchair is equipped and, for some manual chair riders, how easily you can tip back on two wheels.

Certain wheelchair features aid in negotiating curbs and other obstacles. Larger, air-filled wheels and casters go over curbs more easily than hard, smaller wheels. Shock absorbers or an independent suspension system also help in getting over changes in surface level. See Chapter 12, *Tires, Casters, and Suspension Systems*, for more information. For power chair users, Chapter 8, *Power Chair Decisions*, contains a discussion of front-wheel drive systems, a design some people tout as significantly advantageous for climbing curbs.

The ANSI/RESNA testing standards include a specification for maximum obstacle height. Tests are performed considering approach angle, forward or backward movement, and whether or not the chair is in motion as it approaches the obstacle.

For manual chair riders, moving the chair over obstacles can often be accomplished with wheeling skill, using the wheelie technique— tipping back on the two main wheels. Occupational/physical therapists will teach this technique to chair riders they feel have sufficient strength and balance. The chair will need to be properly adjusted so that the axle is not too far forward, which makes the chair tip over backward too easily.

Knowing how to do a wheelie is an important tool that adds to independence. Wheelies make it possible to wheel up or down (jump) curbs. A highly skilled wheeler can hop up curbs that are several inches high. Some riders can even wheel down a series of steps, assuming each one is wide enough to stop on and check their balance. In some cities or buildings, skill at doing wheelies can mean the difference between controlling your own mobility, going well out of your way to find a ramp, or having to be helped.

Wheelies can help even when there is a ramp or curb cut. When you approach a ramp going upward, a good push at the base just before the incline will give you momentum to get started up the ramp, saving you much energy. It is also helpful to do a slight wheelie so that your casters land on the ramp rather than having to raise the front of the chair up. Likewise, if you must wait for a light before crossing the street at a curb cut, don't go down the curb cut until your way is clear. That way, you can use the momentum of going down the curb to help you get back up the crown of the street. Use whatever downhill energy you can, rather than wasting it and having to push uphill with your own power. Doing a slight wheelie as you go down the curb cut will help you use your momentum to get up the rise in the street. Techniques like this take some practice, and of course depend on your strength and balance. If you are still working with a therapist, you can discuss developing these skills.

Another advantage of the wheelie is that it can give you an opportunity to change your position. Sitting for long periods of time gets uncomfortable, since the human body is not made for the sitting posture and needs variety. Doing a wheelie changes the pressures on the spine and allows muscles of the upper body to relax, since the back of the chair is now carrying more of your weight. This is similar in principle to what a recline system does.

I'm fond of tipping back against a wall and putting my brakes on because I find the change in posture to be a great relief.

Wheelie expertise offers purely recreational opportunities as well. If you can't resist the urge to show off a little in your wheelchair, doing wheelies is one of the best ways. While he might appear to balance precariously, a properly trained chair rider has great control doing a wheelie. (This is assuming he isn't trying to show off excessively. Pushing that envelope can lead to embarrassing spills.) Rather than teetering on the edge of falling, the wheels are used to control balance by easily managed forward or backward movements. It's just a matter of getting the feel of it. And while you're at it, "popping" a wheelie with a child in your lap is one of the finer pleasures of life on wheels. (Add an optional whinny sound of a horse, if you like.)

Zen wheeling

As you may know, Zen Buddhism is a practice in which you bring your full attention into the present moment. We all spend much of our thoughts reviewing the past or planning the future. It is very difficult to keep our focus on the absolute present.

What does Zen Buddhism have to do with using a wheelchair, you ask? Wheeling can be like a Zen meditation exercise. It is an opportunity to observe the forces at play right *now*—what is commonly referred to as "mindfulness." The principle of mindfulness can be applied to your wheelchair with a technique that could be called Zen Wheeling.

For instance, riders often encounter very tight spaces. The more present (that is, attentive and patient) you are, the less likely you are to bump into one side or the other, jam a finger, or damage your chair in the process.

Similarly, when you are wheeling along a sidewalk, the downhill wheel needs to be pushed a bit harder, or the joystick pulled a bit to the side to keep you on a straight line. The more aware you are of these sometimes subtle forces at play on you or your chair, the more accurately you can respond with just the right amount of effort at the right time to keep yourself traveling on a steady path. The better you observe the cracks, potholes, slopes at doorways, metal plates, and various other features of the terrain on a sidewalk, the better you can make the fine adjustments in wheeling that they require of you, thereby avoiding bumping into something or having to make a sudden movement because you are thrown off your intended path.

When there is a slight rise in a section of concrete, you will want to give a little extra push to raise the front casters very slightly over it, or slow your power chair just a bit as you approach, then accelerate over it. You can also use your body weight, gently pushing against the back of the chair to slightly lift weight from the casters.

When you are pushing a manual chair up a slope, use it as an opportunity to simply take your time, to really feel the forces you are working against. You can waste a lot of effort if you try to go fast, maintain a consistent speed, or wheel in a straight line. But if you use your arms fluidly with the shoulders, apply your upper-body weight as your balance allows, and note the subtle changes in sideways slope, you can find wheeling uphill is actually a calming experience. Sometimes you will even need to come to a stop as you reposition your arms for the next push. The climb will be good exercise, and it will seem that you got up that slope pretty fast exactly because you stopped worrying about how long it was going to take.

When you pay attention, and as you gain a second-nature sense of your chair as an extension of your body, you will be amazed at the kind of sensitivity to your surroundings you can develop. For example, you will find that you are able to judge curb heights or the spaces between cars in a parking lot by fractions of an inch.

It's a fact that both manual and power chair riders develop a certain elegance in the way they move in their chairs. The relationship of your awareness to your terrain, and your sense in your body of what you feel through your chair, is exactly the kind of integral experience taught by Zen masters. Wheeling with mindfulness will preserve your energy, reduce stress, and protect you from the chance of an accident. You might even find that the quality of attention to other aspects of your life will improve.

Conclusion

ALL THE CHOICES YOU HAVE to make can seem overwhelming if you are getting wheels for the first time—and understandably so. But take heart.

First of all, your therapist, the supplier, and the facts of your condition and lifestyle will very quickly narrow these choices down to a much more manageable number. As you read this book, you probably were able to tell right away whether many of these features applied to you or not. The most important thing to realize is that identifying the wheelchair best suited for you is a process that is worth your time and patience.

The array of choices exists exactly because the market for wheelchairs has been expanding for a lot of exciting reasons:

- People are surviving into older age thanks to better health awareness and treatment.

- Medicine is saving the lives of many who would have died.

- Social evolution is beginning to recognize that living with a disability is simply another aspect of human diversity—not a condition that makes a person less human. We recognize that we can live quite fully, even without the complete use of our legs or arms.

Exciting research is being conducted that will lead to further improvements and new ideas in wheelchair design. At the University of Pittsburgh Human Engineering Research Laboratories, Dr. Michael Boninger, together with Dr. Rory Cooper and their team, is using technology to learn more about the interaction between chair and user, and how the impact of chair use affects the human body. One of their developments is the SmartWheel, a laboratory device that provides information about the forces exerted on wrists, arms, and shoulders when a rider pushes his wheels. This information is used to find more effective, less stressful pushing techniques as well as to aid in creating chair designs that will reduce strain and injury. Among many other innovations, these researchers are investigating manual wheelchairs that incorporate gears and power assistance. An exciting current project is a joystick for power chair users who don't have sufficient range of motion to operate a conventional joystick.

Underlying the expanding choices in wheelchair selection, the interest in research, and the ongoing improvements in chair design is the fact that people with disabilities are insisting on control over their own lives. They are willing to explore what is possible on wheels in many new ways, and want to avail themselves of modern materials and technologies. Having the right wheels makes a world of difference in a person's life. It has never before been possible to achieve the degree of comfort and activity available today. You have the opportunity to make choices that will make a tremendous difference in the quality of your life on wheels.

Manual Chair Features and Options

Type of frame
___ Rigid
___ Folding

Chair weight
___ As light as possible
___ May want options that add weight

Cushion
___ Foam
___ Gel
___ Air/dry floatation
___ Urethane honeycomb
___ Alternating pressure
___ Positioning system

Seat width
___ As narrow as possible
___ Allow for thick clothing

Seat depth
___ Optimal support
___ Allow for deep back

Seat height
___ Minimum height
___ Higher than minimum

Seat angle
___ Parallel to ground
___ Seat dump/squeeze

Back support
___ Sling back alone
___ With tension-adjustable straps
___ With lumbar support
___ Deep upholstery rigid back
___ Customized back

Back height
___ Higher
___ Lower
___ Adjustable

Back angle
___ Upright
___ Somewhat reclined

Push handles

___ Prefer to have

___ Prefer not to have

Footrests

___ Fixed (rigid chairs)

___ Swingaway

___ Tight hanger angle

___ Open hanger angle

___ Tapered hangers

___ Single footplate

___ Separate footplates

___ Fixed footplate angle

___ Adjustable footplate angle

___ Heel loops

___ Calf strap

___ Elevating footrest

Wheels

___ Optimal diameter

___ Spokes

___ Molded

___ Axle toward back

___ Axle more forward

___ Quick-release axle

___ Camber

___ No camber

Handrims

___ Optimal size for stroke

___ Anodized coating

___ Plastic coating

___ Foam coating

___ Powder coating

___ Knobs

Wheel locks

___ Standard

___ Undermount

___ Hill holders

___ Extensions

___ None

Tires

___ Pneumatic

___ Knobby

___ Thin-profile

___ Solid rubber

___ Rubber insert

___ Foam-filled

Casters

___ Pneumatic (larger)

___ Solid rubber

___ Plastic

Anti-tippers

___ Prefer to have

___ Prefer not to have

Suspension

___ Rear-wheel

___ Four-wheel

___ Casters

___ None

Armrests

___ Short

___ Long

___ Lock-down

___ Flip-up

___ Swingaway tube

___ None

Clothing guards

___ Integrated into armrest

___ Cloth

___ Plastic

___ None

Notes:

Power Chair Features and Options

Placement of wheel drive
___ Front-wheel drive
___ Rear-wheel drive
___ Mid-wheel drive

Type of drive
___ Direct
___ Belt

Control system
___ Joystick
___ Breath control
___ Chin control
___ Head control
___ Voice control

Control settings
___ Maximum speed desired
___ User-programmable
___ Acceleration/deceleration
___ Vibration sensitivity
___ Service diagnostics

Batteries
___ Gel cell
___ Wet cell
___ Group 22 size
___ Group 24 size
___ Group 27 size

Battery charger
___ For battery size and type
___ Switch mode

Chair weight
___ As light as possible
___ Heavier okay for needed options

Cushion
___ Foam
___ Gel
___ Air/dry flotation
___ Urethane honeycomb
___ Alternating pressure
___ Positioning system
___ Custom-engineered

Seat width

___ As narrow as possible

___ Allow for thick clothing

Seat depth

___ Optimal support

___ Accommodate positioning
  system

Seat height

___ Minimum

___ Higher than minimum

___ Elevating

Seat angle

___ Parallel to ground

___ Seat dump

___ Tilt system

Back support

___ Rigid back

___ Wraparound back

___ Lateral supports

___ Customized

___ Headrest

Back height

___ Minimum height

___ Higher than minimum

___ Adjustable

Back angle

___ Upright

___ Somewhat reclined (fixed)

___ Recline system

___ Tilt system

Push handles

___ Prefer to have

___ Prefer not to have

Footrests

___ Fixed

___ Swingaway

___ Tight hanger angle

___ Open hanger angle

___ Single footplate

___ Separate footplates

___ Fixed footplate angle

___ Adjustable footplate angle

___ Heel loops

___ Calf strap

___ Elevating footrest

___ Integrated platform

Wheels

___ Large

___ Small

___ Spokes

___ Molded

___ Axle toward back

___ Axle more forward

___ Quick-release axle

Wheel locks
___ User operated
___ Assistant operated
___ Both

Tires
___ Pneumatic
___ Large balloon pneumatics
___ Solid rubber
___ Rubber insert
___ Foam-filled

Casters
___ Pneumatic (larger)
___ Solid rubber (smaller)

Anti-tippers
___ Integrated in frame
___ Removeable
___ None

Suspension
___ Rear-wheel
___ Casters
___ Four-wheel
___ None

Armrests
___ Short
___ Long
___ Lock-down
___ Flip-up
___ Molded

Clothing guards
___ Integrated in armrest
___ Optional

Notes:

Resources

Publications

Accent On Living
P.O. Box 700
Bloomington, IL 61702
1-800-787-8444

A general-interest disability magazine.

Disabled Dealer Magazine
1-800-272-6112
Email: *disdeal@aol.com*

Advertises used vehicles and chairs. Includes display advertising and a classified section. Ask for contact information for the regional franchise nearest you.

A Guide to Wheelchair Selection:
How to Use the ANSI/RESNA Wheelchair Standards to Buy a
Wheelchair
Available from the Paralyzed Veterans of America
801 Eighteenth Street, N.W.
Washington D.C. 20006
1-800-424-8200

Written for consumers, a guide to the various tests and criteria involved in the ANSI/RESNA standards for wheelchair makers.

Mainstream Magazine
687 Highland Avenue
P.O. Box 370598
San Diego, CA 92137
http://www.mainstream-mag.com

A general-interest disability magazine.

Med-Sell
10556 Combie Road #6219
Auburn, CA 95602
(916) 272-2071
http://www.nccn.net/~medsell

A newsletter with ads (including a classified section) for new and used medical equipment.

New Mobility Magazine
23815 Stuart Ranch Road
P.O. Box 8987
Malibu, CA 90265
1-800-543-4116
http://www.newmobility.com

A general-interest disability magazine.

Paraplegia News
Paralyzed Veterans of America
801 Eighteenth Street, NW
Washington, D.C. 20006
(202) 872-1300
Email: *pvapub@aol.com*

Published by the Paralyzed Veterans of America for its members and non-member subscribers, it covers a wide range of general-interest disability topics.

Wheelchair Access and News
Wheelchair Access, Inc.
P.O. Box 12
Glenmoore, PA 19343
(610) 942-3266
http://www.waccess.org/

A web site and newsletter with information on wheelchairs, vans, accessible homes, services, and resources.

Internet resources

Following are a selection of web sites and Internet discussion groups that deal with wheelchair and disability information. You can also search the Internet with the keyword "wheelchair" to find more/updated information.

To participate in discussion groups, only an email address is required. One subscribes to such a list, and all messages are sent to all members of the group. Often it is possible to request a digest, in which only one file is received with a full day's discussion.

AbleData
http://www.abledata.com

Wheelchair information.

Amputee Discussion Group
Send to: *amputee@maelstrom.stjohns.edu*
In message area: *subscribe amputee [your name]*
disAbility Resources

Jim Lubin's disAbility Information and Resources
http://www.eskimo.com/~jlubin/disabled/

A comprehensive listing of disability-related sites.

The Boulevard disability product listings
http://www.blvd.com/

HandiRide Discussion Group
Send to: *handiride-l-request@handinet.org*
In message area: *subscribe*

Focused on "technology, transportation, and access for persons with mobility impairments."

Mobility Discussion Group
Send to: *mobility@maelstrom.stjohns.edu*
In message area: *subscribe mobility [your name]*

A coffeehouse format for people with disabilities; open to discussion of all topics.

Muscular Dystrophy Discussion Group
Request information from: *MD-List-Owner@Basix.com*

Polio Discussion Group
Send to: *polio@maelstrom.stjohns.edu*
In message area: *subscribe polio [your name]*

University of Alabama at Birmingham
http://www.spinalcord.uab.edu

A comprehensive database of disability documents, services, and web links. UAB is known for being the keeper of disability statistics.

Dr. Boninger's web site at University of Pittsburgh
http://www.pitt.edu/~rstherl

University of St. John's listserv index list
http://maelstrom.stjohns.edu/archives/index.html

Includes many medical and disability-related discussion lists, available by email subscription.

Manufacturers

21st Century Scientific, Inc.
4915 Industrial Way
Coeur d'Alene, ID 83814
(208) 667-8800

Power wheelchairs, extra-wide models for large users. Tilt and elevator options.

Advantage Bag Company
22633 Ellinwood Drive
Torrance, CA 90505
1-800-556-6307

Carrying packs for wheelchairs and scooters.

A.G.C.I. Handelsges m.b.H.
Hans-Mauracherstr. 8
Graz, A.8044
Austria
011-43-316-393106
Email: *sbreisach@sime.com*

Manual chairs for outdoor use, including a model for playing golf.

American Medical Technologies
160 Lee Street
Canton, GA 30140
1-800-700-8009

Elevating power wheelchair; tilt and recline systems.

Amigo Mobility International
6693 Dixie Highway
Bridgeport, MI 48722
1-800-248-9130
http://www.amigo.com

Scooters.

Axess
2421 South Westgate Road
Santa Maria, CA 93455
(805) 922-1426
http://www.axessmed.com

Makes the Front Runner carrying basket system.

Bodycare, Inc.
315 Gilmer Ferry Road
Ball Ground, GA 30107
1-800-858-9888

Positioning systems.

Broda Seating
P.O. Box 33046, General P.O. Station
Detroit, MI 48232
1-800-668-0637

Manual wheelchairs.

Bruno Independent Living Aids, Inc.
1780 Executive Drive, P.O. Box 84
Oconomowoc, WI 53066
1-800-882-8183
http://www.bruno.com

Scooters.

Cascade Designs
4000 1st Avenue South
Seattle, WA 98134
1-800-827-4548
http://www.cascadedesigns.com

Cushions.

Colours
1591 South Sinclair Street
Anaheim, CA 92806
1-800-892-8998
http://www.coloursbypermobil.com

Manual lightweight wheelchairs, including the Boing rear suspension chair, and sport models for racing, rugby, and more.

Crown Therapeutics/Roho
100 Florida Avenue
Belleville, IL 62221
1-800-851-3449
http://www.rohoinc.com

Air flotation cushions. The Quadtro allows individual inflation of four quadrants.

D&D Technologies
34844 Stewart Drive
Romulus, MI 48174
(313) 942-1875

Power chair charging accessory. Possible to charge from power outlet in a car or van. Produces AC power to plug in televisions, radios, etc.

D. A. Schulman
7701 Newton Avenue North
Brooklyn Park, MN 55444
(612) 561-2908

Alternating pressure cushions.

Damaco, Inc.
5105 Maureen Lane
Moorpark, CA 93021
1-800-432-2434
Email: *damacoinc@aol.com*

Portable power wheelchair.

Diestco Manufacturing Company
P.O. Box 6504
Chico, CA 95927
1-800-795-2392
http://www.diestco.com
Email: *info@diestco.com*

Wheelchair accessories, lap trays, weather shields, cup holders, etc.

Electric Mobility
1 Mobility Plaza
Sewell, NJ 08080
1-800-662-4548
http://www.emobility.com

Scooters.

ErgoAir
131 D.W. Highway, #326
Nashua, NH 03060-5245
1-800-559-9856
http://www.ergoair.com
Email: *ergoair@empire.net*

Alternating pressure wheelchair cushions.

Everest & Jennings
3601 Rider Trail South
Earth City, MO 63045
1-800-235-4661, 1-800-708-9601

A full line of manual and power wheelchairs, tilt and recline systems, and cushions.

Falcon Rehabilitation Products, Inc.
4404 East 60th Avenue
Commerce City, CO 80022
1-800-370-6808
http://www.falconrehab.com

Power/standing wheelchairs, tilt and recline systems. Emphasizes narrow profile for improved access.

Flofit Medical
5455 Spine Road
Boulder, CO 80301
1-800-356-2668
http://www.flofitmed.com
Email: flofit@flofitmed.com

Foam and foam/gel wheelchair cushions.

Freedom Designs
2241 Madera Road
Simi Valley, CA 93065
1-800-331-8551
http://www.freedomdesigns.com

Manual wheelchairs, reclining systems, custom positioning systems.

Frog Legs
P.O. Box 564
Vinton, IA 52349
(319) 373-9393

Caster fork accessory with shock absorption.

Gendron Inc.
P.O. Box 197
Archbold, OH 43502
1-800-537-2521

Manual wheelchairs, including models for obese users.

Grant Airmass
986 Bedford Street
Stamford, CT 06905
1-800-243-5237
http://www.grantairmass.com
Email: *grant@grantairmass.com*

Alternating pressure cushions.

Hatch Gloves
1656 Walter Street
Ventura, CA 93003
1-800-642-0224
http://www.hatch-gloves.com

Protective gloves designed for quadriplegic chair users.

Heelbo
1134 North Homan Avenue
Chicago, IL 60651
1-800-323-5444

Body-positioning jackets and belts.

Hoveround Personal Mobility
2151 Whitfield Industrial Way
Sarasota, FL 34243
1-800-771-6565
http://www.hoveround.com

Mid-wheel and rear-wheel drive power wheelchairs.

Invacare Corporation/PinDot
899 Cleveland Street
Elyria, OH 44036
1-800-333-6900
http://www.invacare.com

Manual and power wheelchairs, cushions and positioning systems.

Iron Horse Productions
2624 Conner Street
Port Huron, MI 48060
1-800-426-0354

High-endurance, four-wheel suspension manual wheelchairs.

Jay Medical (Sunrise)
P.O. Box 18656
Boulder, CO 80309-1656
1-800-648-8282
http://www.sunrisemedical.com

Gel cushions, wheelchair backs.

Kuschall of America
708 Via Alondra
Camarillo, CA 93012-8713
1-800-654-4768

Manual wheelchairs.

Lark of America
P.O. Box 1647
Waukesha, WI 53187
1-800-446-4522

Scooters.

LDC Corp./Lifestand
780-B2 Primos Avenue
Folcroft, PA 19032
1-800-782-6324
http://www.blvd.com/lifestand/index.html
Email: *dallery@msn.com*

Standing manual wheelchairs.

Ken McRight Supplies
7456 South Oswego
Tulsa, OK 74136
(918) 492-9657

"Bye-Bye Decubiti" inflatable wheelchair cushions.

Matrix USA
1815 North Capitol Avenue
Indianapolis, IN 46202
1-800-253-6217
http://www.concentric.net/~matrixx

Customizable cushioning, positioning frame.

MK Battery
1640 Stadium View
Anaheim, CA 92806
1-800-824-5027
http://www.mkbattery.base.org
Email: *mkbattery@mindspring.com*

Wheelchair batteries.

Morgan Technology, Inc.
2230 Wisconsin Avenue
Downers Grove, IL 60515
1-800-906-5483

"Microlite" manual wheelchairs.

National Power Chair
2642 Commerce Boulevard
Mound, MN 55364
1-800-444-3528
Email: *npc@bitstream.net*

Power wheelchairs.

New Hall's Wheels
P.O. Box 380784
Cambridge, MA 02238
(617) 628-6546
http://www.tiac.net/users/newhalls

Customized lightweight manual and sport chairs.

Orthofab
2160 De Celles
Quebec, Quebec G2C 1X8
Canada
(418) 847-5225

Power wheelchairs.

Otto Bock Reha
3000 Xenium Lane North
Minneapolis, MN 55441-2661
1-800-962-2549
http://www.ottobock.com
Email: *ottobockus@aol.com*

Manual wheelchairs, cushions.

Paraglide Sports, Inc.
12001 31st Court North
St. Petersburg, FL 33716
(813) 573-1010

Lightweight manual wheelchairs.

Pegasus Airwave
5300 Broken Sound Boulevard
Boca Raton, FL 33487
(561) 989-9898
http://www.pegasus-airwave.com

Alternating pressure cushions.

Permobil
6B Gil Street
Woburn, MA 01801
(781) 932-9009
Email: *permobil@aol.com*

Power/standing wheelchairs.

Pride Health Care
182 Susquehanna Avenue
Exeter, PA 18643
1-800-800-8586
http://www.pridehealth.com

Power wheelchairs and scooters.

Quickie Designs/Sunrise Medical
2842 Business Park Avenue
Fresno, CA 93727
(209) 292-2171
http://www.sunrisemedical.com

Manual and power wheelchairs, sport chairs, Jay cushions, Soneil SuperCharger battery chargers.

Ranger All Season Corp.
P.O. Box 132
George, IA 51237
1-800-225-3811
http://www.rangerallseason.com

Scooters and accessories.

Span-America Medical Systems
P.O. Box 5231
Greenville, SC 29662
1-800-888-6752

Wheelchair cushions.

Stand-Aid of Iowa, Inc.
P.O. Box 386
Sheldon, IA 51201
1-800-831-8580
http://www.inmax.com/standaid
Email: *standaid@connect.com*

Roll-Aid converts a manual chair to a power chair.

Sun Metal Products, Inc.
2156 N. Detroit Street
P.O. Box 1508
Warsaw, IN 46581-1508
(219) 267-3281

An assortment of wheels, casters, rims, and axles for wheelchairs.

Supracor
2050 Corporate Court
San Jose, CA 95131-1753
1-800-787-7226
http://www.supracor.com

Honeycomb-type cushions.

Teftec
6929 Old Spring Branch Road
Spring Branch, TX 78070
(210) 885-7588
Email: *teftec@teftec.com*

All-terrain power wheelchairs.

Unishape Adaptive Positioning
1630 30th Street, Suite 202
Boulder, CO 80301
(303) 443-8348

Wheelchair cushions.

Wells Lamont Technologies, Inc.
140 Cypress Station, Suite 207
Houston, TX 77090
1-800-642-5012

Push-Ease wheelchair gloves.

Wheelcare, Inc.
3883-E Via Pescador
Camarillo, CA 93012
(805) 383-4477

Power wheelchairs and conversion kit, scooters.

Wheelchairs of Kansas
204 West 2nd Street
P.O. Box 320
Ellis, KS 67637
1-800-537-6454
Email: *whcharks@pld.com*

Power chairs for obese users.

Bibliography

Axelson, Peter, Jean Minkel, and Denise Chesney. *A Guide to Wheelchair Selection: How to Use the ANSI/RESNA Standards to Buy a Wheelchair*. Washington, D.C. 1-800-424-8200, (202) 872-1300.

Davies, Brooks. "Buying a Power Wheelchair." *New Mobility* (February 1997): 64.

Gullett, Wayne. "Chair Checkup." *Paraplegia News* 51, no. 5 (May 1997): 41.

Hockenberry, John. *Moving Violations*. New York: Hyperion Publishers, 1995. 367 pages. ISBN 0-7868-6078-2.

Hollicky, Richard. "Countdown to Comfort." *Paraplegia News* 51, no. 6 (June 1997): 14.

Maddox, Sam. "Front- and Mid-Wheel Drive: A New Era Arrives for Power Chairs." *New Mobility* (January 1998).

"Resource Guide to Seating and Positioning." *Mainstream Magazine* (November 1996).

Shapiro, Joseph P. *No Pity: People with Disabilities Forging a New Civil Rights Movement*. New York: Times Books, 1993. 382 pages. ISBN 0-8129-2412-6.

Vogel, Bob. "Powering Your Chair: Battery Basics." *New Mobility* (September 1996): 59.

Contributors

Russell G. Anderson, Michael Boninger, M.D., Chris Bourne, Doe Cayting, Jeff Ewing, Jody Greenhalgh, O.T.R., Bob Hall, Warren King (Vice President, Mobility On Wheels), Richard Kratt, Shawn Logan, Kimber Mangiafico, Anet Mconel (Internet alias: AMARIS), Stan Melton, Maureen Pranghofer, Marjie Smith, Karl Ylonen.

Index

A

acceleration, of power chairs, 75, 81
access, home, 42–43, 76, 101
accessories, 133–34
active riders, 3, 43–44. *See also* sport
      chairs; travel
advisors, 32–35. *See also* dealers;
      therapists
air–filled tires, 113–15, 117
ANSI (American National Standards
      Institute), 40, 88, 101, 145
anti–tippers, 117–18
appearance of chair
    manufacturers' attention to, 12,
        17, 18
    not most important feature, 45
    reduces emphasis on disability,
        2, 6, 57, 106
    streamlined in rigid–frame,
        56–57
    See also self–image
armrests, 128–31
axle, adjustable, 8, 46–47, 65–66, 100

B

back support, 70, 103–106
backs, 103–107. *See also* reclining
      backs; tilt feature
back–up chair, 48

batteries, 84–87
belt drive, 77–78, 83–84
brakes, hand, 69–71, 137, 138
braking
    distance, of manual chairs, 64
    with handrims, 68
    on power chairs, 81, 82, 83–84
breath controls on power chairs, 79

C

calf supports, 110
camber, 62, 66–67
case manager, 24
casters, 115–17
    adjusting, 47
    customized angle and height, 8
    maintenance, 137–38
catalog, buying from, 45–46
charger, battery, 86–87
chin controls for power chairs, 79–80
choices, overwhelming, 30, 41–42, 149
clothing guards, 131–32
consultation with dealer and thera-
      pist, 35–37, 42–44. *See*
      also dealers; therapists
control systems for power chairs,
      79–84
cost of chair, 20. *See also* funding
cushions, 53, 89–96

cushion types
    air/dry flotation, 92–93
    alternating pressure, 95–96
    foam, 90–91, 94
    gel, 91–92
    urethane honeycomb, 93–94
    See also positioning systems

D, E

dealers, wheelchair, 33–35
    and economic incentives, 13–14,
        35
    experience with large manufact-
        urers, 12
    knowledge limitations, 14, 34–35
    and production schedule, 15
    and servicing chair, 13, 46, 48,
        135
    and small manufacturers, 15
delivery time, 14–15, 18, 37–38
direct drive, 77–78, 83–84
doctors, 22–23, 32–33
dump, seat, 64–65, 101–103

F

fly–fishing, chair for, 8
foam–filled tires, 115
folding chairs
    development of, 4
    footrests, swingaway, 110
    maintenance, 139
    motorized, 16
    stability on uneven surfaces, 61
    versus rigid–frame, 56–63
    See also manual chairs
footplates, 109–10, 112
footrests, 109–12
    angle of 110–12, 116

elevating, 122
ground clearance, recommended,
    101
heel loops, 110, 137, 139
and home access, 42–43, 44
seat height determined by, 100
front–wheel drive, 72–73, 77
funding, 20–29
    advocacy, when denied, 21–23, 26
    alternative sources of, 24, 28–29
    case manager, 24
    contact person, 23–24, 25
    dealer, insurer may specify, 35
    and dealer knowledge, 34, 35

G

golf, chair for, 16–17
guards, clothing, 131–32

H

Hamilton, Marilyn, 5–6, 7, 10
hand brakes, 69–71, 137, 138
handles, push, 107–108
handrims, 68–69
hangers, footrest, 110–12
head controls for power chairs, 79–80
head supports, 126–27
heel loops, 110, 137, 139
height, seat–to–floor, 42–43, 64–65,
    100–101, 123
history of chair design, 3–10
home access, 42–43, 101

I, J, K

illness, progressive, 31–32, 53, 72
insurance, private, 21, 24–26. *See
    also* funding
Internet resources, 161–62

safety (*continued*)

setting controls for power chairs, 81

speed, maximum in power chair, 82–84

tilt feature and front–wheel drive, unstable, 73

tipping, 73–76, 117–18, 123

when transferring to/from chair, 43, 129, 132

wheel locks, 69–71

See also maintenance

salesperson. *See* dealers

scooters, 52–55

seats, 97–103

angle of, 64–65, 101–103

depth of, 99–100

height of, 42–43, 64–65, 100–101, 123

width of, 97–99

second–hand chairs, 28–29, 78

selection, benefits of knowledge

confidence in chosen manufacturer, 11

decision making, full participation in, 36–37, 39, 41

home access, ensure optimal, 42–43

lifestyle, optimal chair for, 43–44

lower–priced chair, may find, 23

specifications, ensure correct, 38

selection process, 30–38

advisors, 32–35 (*see also* dealers; therapists)

benefits of right chair, 1, 30, 142–43

consultation, 35–37, 42–44

difficulties of, 30 (*see also* problems when buying chair, possible)

open mind, importance of, 44–45

ordering chair, 37–38

trial chair, 37

selection of wrong chair, consequences of

access limited, 34–35, 42–43, 97–98

expense, additional, 38, 39

lifestyle compromised, 44

medical problems, 22–23, 99

pushing more difficult, 64

replacement, wait for funding, 39

safety issues, 43

self–image

improved with modern design, 6

public view, concern about, 31–32, 50–51, 101, 106, 144

style–awareness, 12, 18, 43

and wheeling style, 143–44

See also appearance of chair

service, finding, 12–13, 18–19. *See also* maintenance

shear, 90, 102, 124–25. *See also* cushions; pressure sores

shock absorbers, 61, 77, 118–19

sideguards, 131–32

sip–and–puff controls, 79–80

solid rubber tires, 114–15, 117

sores. *See* pressure sores

specialized chairs, 8–9, 16–17, 61

speed, maximum, 81, 82–84, 143

spokes, maintenance, 138

sport chairs, 4, 8, 16–17, 61–63, 68

squeeze, seat, 64–65, 101–103

standards for chairs, ANSI/RESNA, 40–41, 88, 145

standing position, chairs for, 7–8, 9, 16–17

suspension systems, 61, 77, 118–19

T

terrain, traversing rough
    caster type, impact of, 116
    chairs made for, 9, 116, 118–19
    frame type, which is best, 61
    front–wheel drive, can make easier, 73
    and home access, 42
    suspension systems for, 118–19

tests done on chairs, 40–41, 88, 145

therapists, occupational and physical, 32–33
    and home access, 42
    funding for chair, help to get, 22–23
    knowledge limitations, 14, 33
    pressure sores, alter cushion for, 91

tilt feature, 8, 73, 120–23. *See also* reclining backs

tipping, risk of, 66, 73–76, 123. *See also* anti–tippers

tires, 113–15, 117, 137–38. *See also* casters; wheels

toe–in/toe–out, wheels angled, 67

travel issues
    parts and service, 12–13, 18–19, 135
    power chair batteries, airplane regulations, 85, 87
    right chair for, 43

trial chair, 37, 45

turning radius, 73–76, 111

U, V

used chairs, 28–29, 78

VA (Veterans' Administration), 28, 40. *See also* funding

vehicles, fitting chairs into, 42–43, 56, 60

Vocational Rehabilitation, 27–28. *See also* funding

W–Z

weight, chair, 63–64, 86

weight control and chair width, 98–99

wheelies, 65–66, 145–47

wheeling style and technique, 142–48

wheel locks, 69–71, 137, 138

wheels
    diameter, 64–65
    maintenance, 137–38
    molded, 65
    placement of, 46, 65–66
    size of, on power chairs, 77
    spoked, 65
    tires, 113–15, 117
    See also casters; handrims

width of chair, 34–35, 77, 97–99
    camber adds to, 66–67
    and home access, 42–43

Zen wheeling, 147–48

About the Author

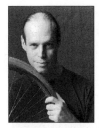

In 1973 when he was 18, Gary fell out of a tree, breaking his spine in mid-back and becoming paraplegic. After missing a term of school, Gary went on to get a B.Arch. from Lawrence Technological University in Southfield, Michigan. He has worked in the computer graphics field managing production departments, starting a desktop services division, and conducting training and presentations. In 1992, Gary developed a repetitive strain injury. After recovering, he began his own ergonomics consulting business, Onsight Technology, which offers training and individual workstation consultation to a wide range of clients in the San Francisco Bay area, where Gary now lives.

Outside work, Gary has been performing music—playing guitar and piano and singing—in local cafés and coffeehouses since he was a teenager. He has also recorded an album of orginial guitar music.

In 1988, a friend introduced him to juggling, and Gary has been hooked ever since. He enjoys the juggling community, the necessity of making mistakes, pushing the envelope of what one is able to do, the Zen experience of staying in the moment, and juggling with others in passing patterns. He has also produced, performed, and emceed at fundraisers and competitions. Through his writing, Gary is interested in helping people make efficient adaptations to using a wheelchair so they can have the best quality of life as quickly as possible. After *Choosing a Wheelchair*, he is working on *Life on Wheels*, which will be published in late 1998.

Photo by Katya Kallsen

Colophon

Patient-Centered Guides are about the experience of illness and disability. They contain personal stories as well as a mixture of practical and medical information.

The pictures on the covers of our Guides reflect the personal side of the information we offer.

The cover of Choosing a Wheelchair was designed by Hanna Dyer and Edie Freedman, using Adobe Photoshop 4.0 and QuarkXpress 3.32. The cover photo is of Gary Karp and was taken by Larry Watson.

The interior layout of this book was created by Edie Freedman and Nancy Priest. The font is Berkeley from the Bitstream foundry. Kristin Murphy did the page makeup using QuarkXPress 3.32. Illustrations were created by Robert Romano using Adobe Photoshop 4 and Macromedia FreeHand 7. This book was copyedited by Lunaea Hougland and proofread by Phylllis Lindsay. Jane Ellin, Madeleine Newell, and Sheryl Avruch performed quality control checks. Carol Wenmoth wrote the index and the colophon.

Permission to reprint photographs in Choosing a Wheelchair has been granted by the following:

The photograph of the SuperLight™ three-wheeled scooter is reprinted by permission of Hal Gutterman of Wheelcare, Inc. The SuperLight™ disassembles in less than a minute, is super lightweight at 83 pounds, and is easy to transport, even in a sub-compact.

The photographs of the Shadow Heat sport chair, Quickie 2 manual folding chair, and J2 Deep Contour back were taken by Keith Seaman of Camerad and are reprinted with his permission.

The photographs of the Action A-4™ rigid-frame manual wheel-chair and the Action Power 9000™ Storm Series® wheelchair are reprinted by permission of Invacare.

The photograph of the Chairman front-wheel drive power chair is reprinted by permission of Goran Udden, president of Permobil.

The photographs of the power chairs with LaBac tilt and recline systems are reprinted by permission of LaBac by Everest & Jennings.

The photograph of the chair back with tension-adjustable straps was taken by Larry Watson of O'Reilly & Associates, Inc.

Patient-Centered Guides™

Questions Answered
Experiences Shared

We are committed to empowering individuals to evolve into informed consumers armed with the latest information and heartfelt support for their journey.

When your life is turned upside down, your need for information is great. You have to make critical medical decisions, often with what seems little to go on. Plus you have to break the news to family, quiet your own fears, cope with symptoms or treatment side effects, figure out how you're going to pay for things, and sometimes still get to work or get dinner on the table.

Patient-Centered Guides provide authoritative information for intelligent information seekers who want to become advocates of their own health. They cover the whole impact of illness on your life. In each book, there's a mix of:

- **Medical background for treatment decisions**
  We can give you information that can help you to intelligently work with your doctor to come to a decision. We start from the viewpoint that modern medicine has much to offer and also discuss complementary treatments. Where there are treatment controversies we present differing points of view.

- **Practical information**
  Once you've decided what to do about your illness, you still have to deal with treatments and changes to your life. We cover day-to-day practicalities, such as those you'd hear from a good nurse or a knowledgeable support group.

- **Emotional support**
  It's normal to have strong reactions to a condition that threatens your life or changes how you live. It's normal that the whole family is affected. We cover issues like the shock of diagnosis, living with uncertainty, and communicating with loved ones.

Each book also contains stories from both patients and doctors — medical "frequent fliers" who share, in their own words, the lessons and strategies they have learned when maneuvering through the often complicated maze of medical information that's available.

We provide information online, including updated listings of the resources that appear in this book. This is freely available for you to print out and copy to share with others, as long as you retain the copyright notice on the print-outs.

http://www.patientcenters.com

Patient-Centered Guides
Published by O'Reilly & Associates, Inc.
Our products are available at a bookstore near you.
For information: **800-998-9938 • 707-829-0515 • info@oreilly.com**
101 Morris Street • Sebastopol • CA • 95472-9902

Other Books in the Series

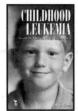

Childhood Leukemia
A Guide for Families, Friends, and Caregivers

By Nancy Keene
ISBN 1-56592-191-7
Paperback, 6 x 9", 539 pages, $24⁹⁵

This complete guide offers detailed and precise medical information for parents that includes day-to-day practical advice on how to cope with procedures, hospitalization, family and friends, school, social, emotional and financial issues, as well as tools to be strong advocates for their child.

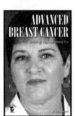

Advanced Breast Cancer
Holding Tight, Letting Go, 2nd Edition

By Musa Mayer
ISBN 1-56592-522-X
Paperback, 520 pages (est.), $19⁹⁵

This updated edition contains new information on medical treatments for metastatic breast cancer. It offers the stories of 40 women and men as they live with metastatic breast cancer, often for many years. The book covers coping with the shock of recurrence, treatment decisions, managing side effects and pain, finding support, family issues, and dealing with emotions.

Your Child in the Hospital
A Practical Guide for Parents

By Nancy Keene & Rachel Prentice
ISBN 1-56592-346-4
Paperback, 5 x 8", 128 pages, $9⁹⁵

This hands-on book provides tips and wisdom that will help make any hospital stay easier. It includes essential information on preparing your child, common procedures, surgery, pain management, feelings and behavior, keeping family life going, the nuts and bolts of hospital records, billing, insurance and how to seek financial assistance.

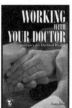

Working With Your Doctor
Strategies for Optimal Health

by Nancy Keene
ISBN 1-56592-273-5
Paperback,: 6 x 9", 350 pages (est.), $15⁹⁵

This is a thorough and useful guide on how to get the greatest care in today's complicated medical world. Topics discussed include how to find the right doctor, communicate clearly, ask about tests and treatments, take action when wronged, and deal with managed care.

Patient-Centered Guides
Published by O'Reilly & Associates, Inc.
Our products are available at a bookstore near you.
For information: **800-998-9938 • 707-829-0515 • info@oreilly.com**
101 Morris Street • Sebastopol • CA • 95472-9902

Here at Patient-Centered Guides we're dedicated to providing the most comprehensive practical, medical and emotional information to readers such as yourself. Please take a moment to fill out the card below so we can learn how to better serve you and others.

We do not sell our mailing list to outside firms.

We'd appreciate hearing from you

Which book did this card come from?

_____

Why did you purchase this book?
❏ I am directly impacted
❏ A family member or friend is directly impacted
❏ I am a health-care practitioner looking for information to recommend to patients and their families
❏ Other _____

How did you first find out about the book?
❏ Recommended by a friend/colleague/family member
❏ Recommended by a doctor/nurse
❏ Saw it in a bookstore
❏ Online
❏ Other _____
❏ *Please send me the Patient-Centered Guides catalog.*

What sources do you use to gather your medical information?
❏ Friends/family   ❏ A library
❏ Your doctor   ❏ Your nurse(s)
❏ Television (which shows?)
❏ Newspapers (which newspapers?)
❏ Magazines (which magazines?)
❏ Newsletters (which newsletters)
❏ The Internet (which newsgroups, mailing lists or Web sites?)
❏ Support Groups (which groups?)
❏ Other _____

What other medical conditions are of concern to you, your family, and community?

_____
_____

Name   Company/Organization (Optional)

Address

City   State   Zip/Postal Code   Country

Telephone   Internet or other email address (specify network)

BUSINESS REPLY MAIL

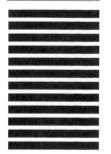